Core Topics in Congenital Cardiac Surgery

Core Topics in Congenital Cardiac Surgery

Edited by

David J. Barron
Birmingham Children's Hospital NHS Trust, United Kingdom

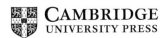

CAMBRIDGE
UNIVERSITY PRESS

University Printing House, Cambridge CB2 8BS, United Kingdom

One Liberty Plaza, 20th Floor, New York, NY 10006, USA

477 Williamstown Road, Port Melbourne, VIC 3207, Australia

314–321, 3rd Floor, Plot 3, Splendor Forum, Jasola District Centre, New Delhi – 110025, India

79 Anson Road, #06–04/06, Singapore 079906

Cambridge University Press is part of the University of Cambridge.

It furthers the University's mission by disseminating knowledge in the pursuit of education, learning and research at the highest international levels of excellence.

www.cambridge.org
Information on this title: www.cambridge.org/9781107034013
DOI: 10.1017/9781139524087

First published 2018

Printed in the United Kingdom by TJ International Ltd. Padstow Cornwall

A catalogue record for this publication is available from the British Library

Library of Congress Cataloging-in-Publication Data
Names: Barron, David J. (David James), editor.
Title: Core topics in congenital cardiac surgery / edited by David J. Barron.
Description: Cambridge, United Kingdom ; New York : Cambridge University Press, 2018. |
Includes bibliographical references and index.
Identifiers: LCCN 2018011857 | ISBN 9781107034013 (hardback : alk. paper)
Subjects: | MESH: Cardiovascular Abnormalities – surgery | Cardiac Surgical
Procedures – methods | Child | Adult
Classification: LCC RD598 | NLM WG 220 | DDC 617.4/12–dc23
LC record available at https://lccn.loc.gov/2018011857

ISBN 978-1-107-03401-3 Hardback

....

Contents

Contents

The colour plates are to be found between pp. 112 and 113

Contributors

David J. Barron FRCS FRCP MD FRCS(CTh)
Birmingham Children's Hospital, United Kingdom

Phil Botha PhD FRCS(CTh)
Birmingham Children's Hospital, United Kingdom

William J. Brawn MD FRACS FRCS
Birmingham Children's Hospital, United Kingdom

Timothy J. Jones MD FRCS(CTh)
Birmingham Children's Hospital, United Kingdom

Natasha Khan MD FRCS(CT)
Birmingham Children's Hospital, United Kingdom

Oliver Stumper MD PhD
Birmingham Children's Hospital, United Kingdom

The Fetal Circulation and Patent Ductus Arteriosus

Timothy J. Jones

Introduction

In contrast to the adult, who is surrounded by air with a changing environmental temperature, the developing fetus is surrounded by amniotic fluid at 37°C. The fetus relies upon the maternal circulation for provision of nutrients, removal of metabolites and respiration, including oxygen supply and carbon dioxide removal. The fetus is a rapidly developing organism, but it exists in a state of relative hypoxia. The developing brain is the most sensitive organ to hypoxia, and the fetal cardiovascular system ensures delivery of the highest oxygenated blood to the brain, whilst blood is distributed to the remaining organs depending on local requirements.

Comparison of the Adult and Fetal Circulations

In health, the adult circulation contains approximately 5 litres (66 mL/kg) of blood, equivalent to 6 to 8 per cent of body weight. Eighty per cent of the circulating volume is in the systemic veins, right side of the heart and pulmonary circulation. The cardiac output is approximately 5 litres/min (~66 mL/kg/min) secondary to a left ventricle contracting 70 times per minute and ejecting a stroke volume of 70 mL with each contraction. Deoxygenated blood returns to the right ventricle, and the entire cardiac output passes via the pulmonary arteries to the lungs for the purposes of gas exchange. Oxygenated blood returns via the pulmonary veins to the left ventricle and systemic circulation. The right and left sides of the heart are separate, and the pulmonary and systemic circulations are in series. The pulmonary circulation is low pressure (25/10 mmHg) compared to the systemic circulation (120/80 mmHg).

In the fetus, gas exchange occurs at the placenta. For oxygenated blood to return to the systemic circulation and deoxygenated blood to the placenta there are several communications or shunts present, and the two circulations are in parallel with both ventricles contributing to the total cardiac output. The fetal circulation is illustrated in Figure 1.1.

The fetal cardiac output is approximately 300 mL/min/kg, with the right ventricle contributing approximately two-thirds of the total cardiac output. The heart rate is 130 to160 beats/min. Approximately 40 per cent of the cardiac output perfuses the placenta and returns to the heart via the umbilical venous

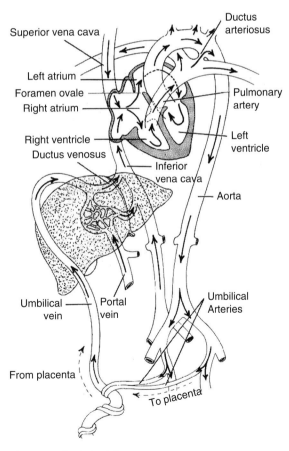

Figure 1.1 Fetal circulation.
Source: From Ganong's Review of Medical Physiology, Twenty-Fourth Edition © 2012 by The McGraw-Hill Companies, Inc

Table 1.1 Oxygen Saturations within the Fetal Circulation

Location	Oxygen saturation (%)
Umbilical veins	80
Ductus venosus	75
Left atrium	70
Ascending aorta	65
Right ventricle	55
Ductus arteriosus	52
Descending aorta	55
IVC (below the ductus venosus)	25
SVC	25

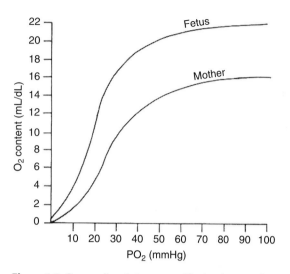

Figure 1.2 Oxygen dissociation curve of fetal and maternal haemoglobin.
Source: From Ganong's Review of Medical Physiology, Twenty-Fourth Edition © 2012 by The McGraw-Hill Companies, Inc

system with an oxygenation saturation of approximately 80 per cent. This is the most highly saturated fetal blood in the circulation. Half this blood supplies the liver, and the rest passes via the ductus venosus to the inferior vena cava (IVC), where it meets the desaturated systemic venous drainage from the lower body. Selective streaming of these two flows minimizes mixing with the well-oxygenated blood from the ductus venosus, which is directed posterior and leftward in the IVC. The blood from the IVC enters the right atrium, and further streaming occurs via the anatomical configuration of the Eustachian valve and the upper margin of the foramen ovale to split the stream of blood into an anterior rightward stream that enters the right atrium and a posterior leftward stream (well-oxygenated ductus venosus blood) to the left atrium. Despite this arrangement, some mixing does occur, but the oxygen saturation of the left atrial blood is approximately 70 per cent (Table 1.1). This blood is ejected by the left ventricle to supply the heart and brain. Desaturated blood returning from the upper body via the superior vena cava (SVC) is directed through the tricuspid valve along with the desaturated blood from the coronary sinus into the right ventricle. This accounts for approximately 60 per cent of the venous return to the heart and explains why the right ventricle contributes to two-thirds of the cardiac output. The right ventricular blood is approximately 55 per cent saturated. Only 8 per cent of the combined ventricular output passes to the pulmonary circulation; the remainder passes directly via the ductus arteriosus to the descending aorta. The pulmonary vascular resistance is very high due to the presence of relatively few arteries and because the lungs are not expanded. The right atrial pressure is higher than the left,

reflecting the greater blood flow through the right atrium. The ductus arteriosus creates little resistance, and the right ventricular and pulmonary artery pressure is 1 to 2 mmHg higher than that of the aorta (55/35 mmHg) and left ventricle (55/2 mmHg).

Fetal Haemoglobin

The maternal arterial blood in the placenta has an oxygen saturation of 80 to 90 per cent. The essential characteristic of fetal haemoglobin is that it has a higher affinity for oxygen than maternal haemoglobin. Fetal haemoglobin (Hb-F) has an oxygen dissociation curve that is displaced to the left compared to adult/maternal haemoglobin (Figure 1.2). This displacement increases the slope of the curve, and consequently, for a given partial pressure of oxygen (PO_2), more HbO_2 is formed. The difference is due to Hb-F binding 2,3-diphosphoglycerate less effectively than maternal Hb. At birth, 80 per cent of the fetal haemoglobin is Hb-F, and this falls to approximately 10 per cent by four months of age.

Changes in Fetal Circulation at Birth

At birth, the pulmonary circulation is established, followed by closure of fetal shunts (Figure 1.3). The placental circulation is interrupted, which increases systemic vascular resistance and decreases IVC return and right atrial filling. There is an increase in oxygen utilization secondary to increased work of breathing

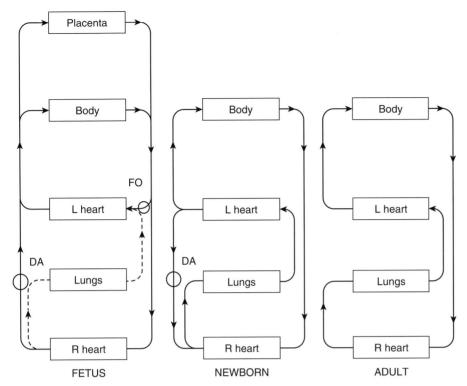

Figure 1.3 Changes in the fetal circulation at birth. *Source:* From Ganong's Review of Medical Physiology, Twenty-Fourth Edition © 2012 by The McGraw-Hill Companies, Inc

which is accompanied by an increase in cardiac output. As the lungs are expanded, oxygen levels increase, and vasodilators including nitric oxide are released. The pulmonary vascular resistance falls to approximately half the systemic values by the first 24 hours of life. There is an eight- to tenfold increase in pulmonary blood flow resulting in increased blood flow to the left atrium. The pressure difference between the right and left atrium is reversed, and this closes the flap valve of the foramen ovale. The ductus arteriosus begins shunting left to right before it begins to constrict due to the production of bradykinin stimulated by increasing oxygenation and the fall in circulating prostaglandins.

Persistent fetal circulation or 'persistent pulmonary hypertension of the newborn (PPHN)' occurs in approximately 0.1 to 0.2 per cent of live births. The usual changes at birth of pulmonary vasodilatation, ductal closure and closure of the foramen ovale do not occur. The pulmonary vascular resistance remains high, even in excess of systemic vascular resistance. This results in decreased blood flow to the lungs, and instead, blood passes from the pulmonary artery via the patent ductus arteriosus to the systemic circulation. This results in a right-to-left shunt. In addition, the right ventricular and right atrial pressures remain elevated and in excess of left atrial pressure. The flap valve of the foramen ovale does not close, and a further right-to-left shunt occurs at atrial level, with blood bypassing the pulmonary circulation. The presence of right-to-left shunts and decreased pulmonary blood flow results in hypoxia.

Patent Ductus Arteriosus

The patent ductus arteriosus (PDA) usually closes in the first month of life. In premature babies, ductal closure may not occur such that 80 per cent of premature babies weighing less than 1,200 g will have a patent duct (PDA). Many of these babies are asymptomatic, but those with a large duct and a significant left-to-right shunt will present in congestive cardiac failure with bounding pulses, continuous murmur and a volume-loaded left ventricle. Initially, the baby is managed with anti-failure medication. A course of indomethacin or ibuprofen can be used to precipitate ductal closure, but if this is unsuccessful, the duct has to be closed surgically, usually via a left lateral thoracotomy. Indomethacin is contra-indicated in patients with renal insufficiency or intra-cranial haemorrhage. The use of these drugs has reduced the need for surgical closure from 30 to 5 per cent of haemodynamically significant ducts.

In larger children (>4 kg), the duct may be occluded using a trans-catheter device.

Morphology. The arterial duct connects the main pulmonary artery with the descending aorta, just distal to the origin of the left subclavian artery. If there is a left aortic arch, it is usually left sided; in right aortic arch, it may be left or right sided. In some conditions, it may be absent or, rarely, bilateral. It varies in length and diameter. The media consists of spirally arranged smooth muscle, and the intima is thicker than the aorta. After birth, the media contracts, thus shortening and occluding the duct. The endothelial layer folds, the subintimal layers proliferate and the duct thus closes permanently within two to three weeks of birth. This process can be delayed by prostaglandins E1 and E2 and prostacyclin.

Pathophysiology. After birth, the pulmonary vascular resistance falls, and there is left-to-right shunting from the aorta to the pulmonary arteries, leading to over-circulation and congestive heart failure.

Presentation

Premature infants with this defect may be ventilator dependent or require long periods of non-invasive ventilation. Many older children may be asymptomatic. Large shunts may present as congestive heart failure early in life.

Procedure. In the United Kingdom, the majority (90 per cent) of surgical PDA ligations are performed in premature neonates. The approach is via left lateral thoracotomy in the fourth intercostal space. Access in the small chest cavity, retracting the congested lung, is limited. The duct is frequently the same size as the descending aorta, and the anatomy of the arch must be clearly defined to prevent inadvertent ligation of the aortic arch. Once defined, the PDA is either ligated with a ligature or with LIGACLIPS according to surgical preference. Encircling with a ligature gives better definition of the anatomy but may carry greater risk of damaging the fragile ductal tissue. There should be immediate improvement in diastolic pressure.

Ligation in older children is now virtually unknown due to the success of interventional device closure. However, if referred an older child the duct will have become a much more rigid structure and surgery may require formal mobilization, transection and over-sewing of the PDA to ensure that there is no residual shunt.

The greatest risk in these fragile babies is haemorrhage, but the incidence is less than 0.5 per cent. Other complications include recurrent laryngeal nerve injury, chylothorax and pneumothorax. Despite being a safe procedure, the 30-day mortality remains relatively high (5 per cent) reflecting the co-morbidities of (what is often) extreme prematurity.

Essentials of Paediatric Cardiopulmonary Bypass

Timothy J. Jones

Introduction

Since its first successful application in 1953, advances in cardiopulmonary bypass (CPB) in conjunction with developments in operative technique and postoperative care have resulted in increasingly complex cardiac surgery being successfully undertaken on younger and smaller children. With mortality rates improving, the focus is now changing to reducing the morbidity associated with paediatric surgery and CPB. The effects of hypothermia, altered perfusion, haemodilution, acid-base management, embolization and the systemic inflammatory response still pose significant problems. Infants and neonates present additional challenges due to their small size, immature organ systems and altered physiology.

Neonatal Physiology

The normal changes in physiology in the first weeks of life, including the reactivity of the pulmonary vasculature, influence both technique and outcome of surgical repair. Pulmonary hypertension, present at birth, decreases to approximately 50 per cent of systemic values within the first 24 to 48 hours of life but takes several weeks to completely resolve. The neonatal myocardium is relatively resistant to ischaemia but has limited functional reserve, being susceptible to increased afterload (systemic and pulmonary vascular resistance). Neonates have a higher metabolic rate requiring higher pump flow rates per kilogram compared to an adult and an impaired thermoregulatory response with greater dependence upon environmental temperature. Variability in heparin and protamine pharmacokinetics and immaturity of the liver may result in a coagulopathy that will be worsened by the presence of cyanosis. Renal perfusion and glomerular filtration are decreased due to increased renal vascular resistance, resulting in impaired sodium, water and acid-base regulation. While humoral and cellular immune factors are present, the immune response is impaired and subnormal. The underlying cardiac pathology or chronic cyanosis may result in the presence of large intra- and extra-cardiac shunts that may need controlling during CPB in order to maintain adequate systemic perfusion and enable visualization of intra-cardiac defects.

The majority of paediatric CPB utilizes haemodilution with moderate hypothermia. In small patients, limited access for surgery and CPB cannulation together with the need to undertake complex repairs with good visibility necessitates periods of deep hypothermic circulatory arrest.

Prime and Haematocrit

Haemodilution during CPB theoretically counterbalances the increase in blood viscosity caused by induced hypothermia, resulting in improved microcirculatory perfusion. In addition, it is associated with less red blood cell aggregation and increased cerebral blood flow velocity. It does, however, reduce clotting factors and also plasma oncotic pressure, enabling fluid to move from the intravascular space into the intracellular space and causing tissue oedema and impaired organ function. The accumulation of fluid is more common in neonates secondary to increased capillary permeability.

The extremes of haemodilution (~10 per cent haematocrit) are associated with impaired oxygen delivery and delayed cerebral recovery following deep hypothermic circulatory arrest (DHCA). Acceptable levels of haematocrit are not yet clearly defined, and they vary between 20 and 30 per cent for neonatal deep hypothermic bypass. Recent work does suggest that higher haematocrits of 30 per cent are probably beneficial to postoperative long-term psychomotor development.

The blood volume of a neonate is around 85 mL/kg, with a 3-kg child having a circulatory volume of approximately 255 mL. A CPB prime volume of 650 to 800 mL will result in a prime-to-blood-volume ratio of 2:1 or 3:1. The priming volume should be kept as small as possible by the utilization of appropriately sized equipment and with correct positioning of the CPB apparatus to avoid unnecessary lengths of tubing. Administration of crystalloid fluids during CPB to maintain an adequate working volume will result in further haemodilution. During CPB, the addition of fluid to the circuit should only be to maintain the minimum safe working volume, and crystalloid volume replacement should be avoided.

The composition of the prime is dictated by the size of the child, the preoperative haemoglobin, the maintenance of colloid oncotic pressure, the surgical procedure and personal preference. Typically for a neonate, the prime may consist of Plasmalyte 148 (30 mL/kg), 1 unit of fresh frozen plasma, heparin (2,500 units), methylprednisolone (20 mg/kg), calcium chloride (2.5 mmol), sodium bicarbonate 8.4 per cent (10 mL), mannitol (0.5 g/kg) and irradiated red blood cells.

With attention to these issues and with the development of paediatric CPB components, it is possible to reduce priming volumes to approximately 300 mL for a 3-kg child. Despite this reduction, maintenance of an intra-operative haematocrit of 30 per cent is likely to require the addition of donor blood. Cardiac surgery and CPB without using blood have been successfully undertaken in children weighing less than 10 kg. To date, there has been no systematic assessment of the safety and efficacy of blood versus blood-free cardiac surgery in children.

Hypothermic Circulatory Arrest and Low-Flow CPB

The decision to use circulatory arrest, low flow, full flow, and high or low perfusion pressures, is based on a combination of patient size, anatomy, surgical procedure, collateral blood flow and personal preference as opposed to predetermined protocols. There is a trend towards less use of deep hypothermia and circulatory arrest with a move towards more physiological parameters.

The optimal temperature for circulatory arrest is thought to be between 14 and 20°C, typically 18°C. Bypass should be continued for at least 20 minutes before the circulation is arrested to ensure uniform cooling. Cyanotic patients with large aorto-pulmonary collaterals have been identified as a group at increased risk of neurological injury associated

with circulatory arrest. Evidence from animal work suggests that the period of cooling should be extended in this group due to delayed brain cooling secondary to reduced cerebral blood flow. The maximum duration of 'safe' DHCA is unknown. It is logical that the period should be as short as possible but long enough to accomplish satisfactory surgical repair. Increased periods of DHCA are associated with increased brain injury. However, the use of a short period of DHCA to quickly complete an accurate reconstruction may be preferable to struggling with poor visibility and leaving the patient with a suboptimal repair.

Circulatory arrest provides good visibility and improved surgical access, but concerns regarding neurological complications have led to the development of alternative techniques particularly during neonatal and infant surgery. The reduction in cerebral metabolic activity during cooling is greater than the reduction in cerebral blood flow and oxygen delivery. Low-flow, low-temperature CPB is based upon this principle. Low-flow CPB when compared to DHCA has been associated with a lower incidence of seizures and improved EEG recovery with better neurology, motor function and language skills. By eight years of age there were no differences between the two groups, but overall neurodevelopmental status for both groups was below expectations. The DHCA group continued to demonstrate lower test scores with regard to motor function and speech.

Circulatory arrest may still be required in small neonates when access is otherwise impossible or if venous return is excessive. In such circumstances, intermittent flow during periods of DHCA produces considerably improved cerebral metabolic recovery. Thus, a period of 60 minutes of DHCA is well tolerated with complete cerebral recovery if divided into 15- to 30-minute intervals by short periods of perfusion, even at low flow.

Alternatives to Deep Hypothermic Circulatory Arrest

DHCA provides good visibility and improved surgical access. However, prolonged periods are associated with an increased incidence of brain injury. Concerns regarding neurological complications have led to the development of alternative techniques, particularly during neonatal and infant surgery.

Intermittent flow during periods of DHCA is one such alternative which results in considerably improved cerebral metabolic recovery. Another approach, particularly useful when working on the aortic arch, is selective antegrade cerebral perfusion and low-flow CPB. There is increasing experience of this technique in adults and children undergoing aortic arch surgery. The technique is readily applicable to paediatric surgery. Following a brief period of circulatory arrest, the aortic arch is opened, and the aortic cannula can be advanced directly into the innominate artery. A modification of this technique is to directly cannulate a Gore-Tex tube anastomosed to the innominate artery. Selective antegrade perfusion may improve neurological outcome, and the technique is relatively easy to perform, but there remains no categorical data to conclude that it is superior to DHCA.

There is increasing evidence that the immature brain is particularly susceptible to injury during CPB; this is exacerbated by the fact that brain development can frequently be delayed in many congenital heart conditions.

Hypothermia and Carbon Dioxide Management

Alpha-Stat or pH-Stat Mode? The optimal management of acid-base and arterial carbon dioxide tensions during CPB has been the focus of much research and debate. During 'alpha-stat' management, intracellular pH, enzymatic activity and perfusion-pressure auto-regulation are preserved. In contrast, during 'pH-stat' management, auto-regulation is lost, and cerebral perfusion is in excess of metabolic demands. The increased cerebral blood flow potentially improves brain cooling with redistribution of blood flow to deep brain structures. pH stat results in lower intracellular pH, which may increase cerebral tissue oxygenation by suppressing cellular function. In addition, the oxygen dissociation curve is displaced to the right, thereby liberating more oxygen to the tissues. There are concerns that suppression of cellular function with pH stat results in delayed cerebral metabolic recovery following hypothermic circulatory arrest. As a result of this evidence, alpha stat is the most widely used technique, but some groups use a strategy of pH stat during cooling with conversion to alpha stat prior to circulatory arrest and subsequent re-warming. Such an approach is believed to enhance cerebral cooling and subsequently improve metabolic recovery. The optimal clinical strategy remains unclear because most of the data come from animal work. In a prospective clinical trial undertaken by a Boston group, the use of a pH-stat strategy throughout in infants undergoing deep hypothermic CPB was associated with lower postoperative morbidity and a shorter time to first EEG activity, supporting the clinical advantages of pH management. In a follow-up study there was no significant difference in development or neurological outcome at one, two or four years between pH-stat or alpha-stat groups.

Ultrafiltration

The increasing use of CPB in the neonatal period with haemodilution has exposed the tendency towards capillary leakage in these patients. In conventional ultrafiltration, an ultrafilter within the bypass circuit is used to shunt some blood from the arterial to the venous sides of the circuit either throughout CPB or during re-warming towards the end of bypass to remove excess water from the combined circuit. In contrast, modified ultrafiltration (MUF) is undertaken during a 10- to 15-minute period immediately after cessation of bypass. The arterial cannula is left in place, and the venous cannulae are removed. Blood flows up the aortic cannula to the ultrafilter inlet and is pumped through the filter at 100 to 150 mL/min. The haemoconcentrated blood from the haemofilter passes to the right atrium via a line from the ultrafilter which is heated and placed through the venous cannulation site into the right atrial appendage. This blood is thus haemoconcentrated and warmed as it flows to the right atrial appendage. Ultrafiltration continues until the patient's haemotocrit is elevated to the desired level. Custom-designed ultrafiltration circuits are now available from many manufacturers.

The use of MUF after CPB is associated with a significant reduction in the rise of total body water, a reduction in blood loss and a reduction in the need for blood transfusion during the early postoperative phase. In addition to raising the haematocrit from approximately 20 to 35, there is an associated rise in cardiac index, no significant change in systemic vascular resistance and a fall in pulmonary vascular resistance over the 15-minute period of ultrafiltration.

Summary

Paediatric CPB is generally a well-tolerated procedure. Significant advances in understanding and technique have enabled complex neonatal cardiac surgery to be routinely undertaken. The diverse cardiac pathologies and surgical techniques require the perfusion strategy to be tailored to each individual patient. An understanding of the principles involved helps to provide the optimal strategy to undertake surgery accurately and maximize patient outcome (see Table 2.1).

Table 2.1 Areas of Controversy and Interest in Paediatric CPB

Miniaturization of bypass circuits
Use of pH-stat strategies or combined strategies
Benefit of selective antegrade cerebral perfusion in arch repair
Greater avoidance of DHCA and trend towards warmer bypass
Role of modified ultrafiltration
Prevalence of underlying brain immaturity in congenital heart disease

Chapter 3

Imaging in Congenital Heart Disease

Oliver Stumper

Introduction

The diagnosis of congenital heart disease is a medical/clinical art that has been supported by vast improvement in imaging techniques over the past four decades. It was only in the early 1980s that two-dimensional cardiac ultrasound became a universally available technique to assess cardiac anatomy and function at the bedside. The first Doppler ultrasound machines with colour flow mapping became available in the mid-1980s. Before then, it was clinical diagnosis with a stethoscope, M-mode scans, chest X-ray and cardiac catheterization. We are now practicing in an era where we can generate real-time non-invasive and free of radiation exposure images of the congenitally malformed heart. These techniques have provided us with very detailed insights into cardiac morphology and function.

To undertake surgical treatment of congenital heart disease in the current era requires a sound understanding of the anatomy, physiology and surgical techniques and, above all, the ability to read and interpret the vast range of imaging information that is generated and provided by cardiologists.

Chest X-rays

It is rare that a plain chest X-ray is diagnostic of congenital heart disease. The traditional signs of a 'ground glass' lung field (obstructed total anomalous pulmonary venous drainage) and figure of three with rip notching (established coarctation) are rarely seen in an era of earlier diagnosis and treatment. Nonetheless, the plain chest X-ray remains a good technique in the assessment of cardiomegaly, associated lung pathology, spinal problems, etc. After all the advances in cardiac imaging, the plain chest x-ray remains one of the most powerful predictors of exercise tolerance.

Cardiac Ultrasound

Trans-thoracic Ultrasound. Two-dimensional cardiac ultrasound has revolutionized the assessment of cardiac structure and function over the past three decades. This is a bedside technique which allows for the comprehensive assessment of virtually all neonates, infants and children with congenital heart disease. Limitations are experienced in adults, as ultrasound waves are hampered by intra-thoracic air and poor trans-thoracic windows. The addition of colour flow imaging (from the mid-1980s) has largely facilitated the rapid recognition of intra-cardiac shunt lesions and valvar dysfunction (stenosis and regurgitation).

Doppler ultrasound added a new dimension to cardiac ultrasound investigation of the heart. By measuring flow velocities across the cardiac valves or any existing shunt lesions, it became possible to quantitate intra-cardiac pressure differences during any particular phase of the cardiac cycle. The Bernouille equation, $\Delta P = 4(V_{max}^2)$, strictly applies for only pulsatile flow and instantaneous pressure gradients. Despite these restrictions, and with an awareness of the limitations, it is an extremely valuable bedside technique to assess intra-cardiac pressure differences and thereby postoperative results. In the assessment of aortic or pulmonary valve stenosis or a pulmonary artery band, it is more reliable to take the mean velocity rather than the peak velocity to calculate pressure gradients.

In the current era, it is possible to assimilate very detailed imaging information on the vast majority of neonatal and infant cases with congenital heart disease to plan surgical intervention. In fact, the quality and detail of the images provided render diagnostic cardiac catheterization superfluous in the majority of cases, other than for the detailed assessment of pre-operative haemodynamics. The exception to this is assessment of the peripheral pulmonary arteries or collateral arteries, which are obscured by the lungs (air) during cardiac ultrasound imaging. In these cases, cardiac catheterization and angiography remain the gold standard.

Trans-oesophageal Ultrasound. This became available for the study of young infants and later also neonates in the early 1990s. It has helped us to better understand and evaluate certain aspects of mostly atrial morphology, pulmonary and systemic venous return and the atrio-ventricular (A-V) valves. In the context of ever-increasing resolution and field of depth of trans-thoracic ultrasound (harmonic and 3D imaging), the advantages of trans-oesophageal ultrasound are frequently absent or just marginal. As trans-oesophageal ultrasound requires general anaesthesia in the young patient population, it is now confined mostly to the intra-operative monitoring of cardiac surgical and interventional cardiac catheterization procedures (Figure 3.1).

Intra-operative Ultrasound. Most patients undergoing congenital cardiac surgery benefit from undergoing a cardiac ultrasound study before leaving the cardiac surgical theatre or, for that matter, before removing the cannulation for cardiopulmonary bypass. This is to rule out any significant residual haemodynamic lesions, which could be addressed during a second bypass run, rather than to experience problems on the intensive care unit, with a long way back to the catheterization laboratory or cardiac theatre.

There are two techniques available for use: intra-operative epicardial ultrasound and trans-oesophageal ultrasound. Each has its strengths and weaknesses. The advantages for epicardial ultrasound are that it can be used in virtually every patient and provides superior information in the assessment of the outflow tracts and the great arteries. AV valves can be assessed in detail, and repeat scans can be conducted at various times during the weaning from bypass process. It is very cost effective and does not distract the anaesthetist. Ideally, scans should be conducted by the operating cardiac surgeon. Such a practice enhances the learning curve and provides immediate feedback. The advantage of trans-oesophageal imaging is the ability to provide continuous monitoring of cardiac function and volume status. However, it is very limited in assessing the outflow tracts, pulmonary arteries, aortic arch and haemodynamic status

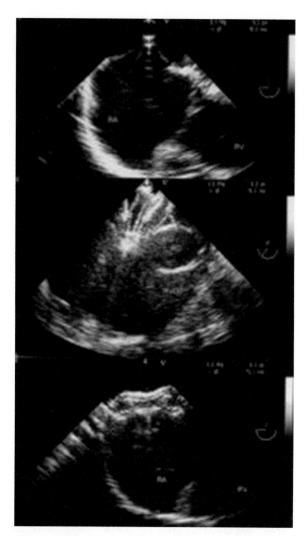

Figure 3.1 Trans-oesophageal imaging of a child with an atrial septal defect undergoing trans-catheter closure. (Above) Four-chamber view with the delivery sheath crossing the atrial septal defect. (Centre) Initial device position is perpendicular to the atrial septum behind the aortic root. (Below) Final device position after release, engaging all the rims of the defect and achieving a flat profile.

using Doppler ultrasound techniques. Also, when it is performed by cardiac anaesthetists, there may be occasions, when a patient is unstable, that there is a conflict between managing ventilation, inotropic support and volume replacement, when, at the same time, detailed high-quality imaging and haemodynamic assessments are required by the surgeon.

The attending paediatric cardiologist should be involved in all discussions of whether to go back on bypass and try to address any potential residual haemodynamic lesions. It is only when the findings of the post-bypass ultrasound studies are discussed within the attending team that the best possible outcome can be achieved.

Quantification of postoperative haemodynamic lesions by intra-operative ultrasound remains an extremely difficult area. In most cases, systemic vascular resistance is increased and cardiac output is decreased. Diffuse shunting across newly placed patches to close ventricular septal defects is common, and an under-filled heart may generate dynamic outflow tract gradients due to persistent hypertrophy and concurrent inotropic support. Surgery is mostly not perfect, and minor residual haemodynamic lesions are the norm. It is the interpretation of the images, the haemodynamics, the understanding of the surgical findings and what has been done during the repair that will guide the team as to what to do next: accept the result, wait and reassess, go back on bypass and revise. These are individual case discussions rather than departmental protocols. In a great number of patients in whom immediate revision on a second period of bypass is being considered, there is a role in obtaining further haemodynamic information. This could entail direct pressure measurements in various cardiac chambers, running multiple saturation measurements so as to quantitate residual shunts, etc. All these techniques have inherent limitations in the immediate post-bypass period and need close discussions to arrive at an agreed plan for further management.

Cardiac Catheterization

Cardiac catheterization and angiography remained the mainstay of cardiac imaging in the 1970s and 1980s but now have been superseded by more modern imaging techniques which do not require general anaesthesia or expose the patient to radiation. Nonetheless, cardiac catheterization remains the gold standard in assessing the pulmonary circulation and in identifying occluded or poorly perfused arteries and capillary vascular beds (Figure 3.2). Its decline in diagnostic imaging has been accommodated by an ever-increasing demand for interventional cardiac catheterization procedures, which constitute 70 to 80 per cent of all procedures in modern laboratories/units. Lesions that are almost exclusively treated with trans-catheter techniques today include pulmonary stenosis, infant and childhood ductus arteriosus and adolescent/adult coarctation (Figure 3.3), as well as the majority of secundum atrial septal defects, childhood aortic stenoses, childhood muscular

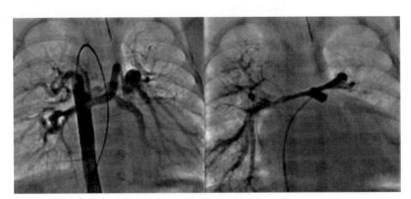

Figure 3.2 Descending aortogram in a child with pulmonary atresia and major aorto-pulmonary collateral arteries (MAPCAs). Following intubation of the left-sided MAPCA, it is possible to enter the native pulmonary artery and obtain selective injections (right).

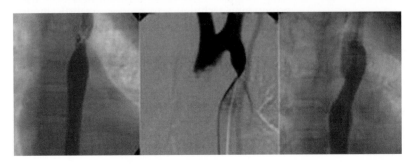

Figure 3.3 Severe coarctation in a teenager. Descending aortogram documents near interruption. Good relief of the obstruction is achieved by placing a covered stent (right).

ventricular septal defects and postoperative pulmonary artery stenoses. There has and always will be a close interface between cardiac catheterization and cardiac surgical programmes and techniques to achieve best patient outcomes. Hybrid cardiac catheter and cardiac surgical procedures will be discussed in more detail in Chapter 23 of this text.

The unequalled ability of cardiac catheterization techniques compared to all other cardiac imaging techniques is the possibility to identify native pulmonary arteries that are no longer perfused. This is of major utility in the management of patients with abnormal pulmonary blood supply, in particular, in those with major aorto-pulmonary collaterals. By crossing the atrial septum and intubating the individual pulmonary veins, a wedge position can be achieved. Angiographic contrast material is then injected into the pulmonary veins and is flushed through by normal saline to delineate the native pulmonary arteries. The clinical benefit of this technique cannot be underestimated in patients with severely hypoplastic or underdeveloped pulmonary artery segments.

Computed Tomography

The development of multi-detector-row computed tomography has rendered CT imaging of the heart a very powerful technique to evaluate even small vessels, including the pulmonary arteries, in young children. Slice thickness of modern equipment is now routinely less than 0.5 mm, and acquisition times for scans are very short. At the same time, the radiation dose exposure during these examinations has been dramatically reduced over the most recent years. Most studies in children compare favourably with the dose exposure during cardiac angiography. In addition, CT studies have the advantage of being non-invasive and not needing general anaesthesia. ECG gating is not required in the assessment of the lung arteries, thereby further reducing time of the study and radiation dose.

The acquired data set can be reconstructed to very detailed three-dimensional models, which can be manipulated further to assess particular areas of interest or to assess the spatial relationship of the intrathoracic vessels to the oesophagus and the bronchial tree. These contributions have made CT a very powerful tool in the assessment of patients with pulmonary atresia and aorto-pulmonary collateral arteries or severely ill children in the intensive care unit.

Cardiac catheterization remains the preferred technique in cases where there is the need for detailed haemodynamic data and those who are likely to require a catheter intervention at the same time.

Magnetic Resonance Imaging

Cardiac MRI imaging using 1.5-T equipment has established itself as a very powerful tool in the comprehensive assessment of older patients with congenital heart disease, in particular, in the growing numbers of adolescent and adult patients. To obtain good images, it is important that the patient can cooperate and perform repeated breath holding. By utilizing detailed departmental protocols, a complete assessment of form, function and haemodynamics can be obtained in the majority of patients. Cardiac MRI has become the gold standard in the assessment of cardiac chamber volumes during the cardiac cycle and calculating blood flow through pulmonary arteries or regurgitant fractions. Late enhancement techniques of the myocardium can be used to assess scarring and infarct size.

The ability to reconstruct 3D data sets, which can be further manipulated, adds further value to the detailed evaluation of a wide range of pre- or postoperative congenital heart disease. As the technique is non-invasive and does not expose the patient to radiation, studies can be repeated over time to assess any progression in observed lesions and to inform clinical management.

Modern cardiac imaging has a number of sophisticated from which tools to choose. Cardiac ultrasound will remain the imaging technique of first choice in the majority of serial investigation and preoperative evaluation of the majority of young children. The next decade will see further developments in the 3D dynamic reconstruction of cross-sectional images, which will further enhance our understanding of the complex anatomies we are dealing with. In time, this will lead to the development of rapid prototyping techniques to produce realistic models to plan future surgical intervention and improve surgical education and training.

Further Reading

Ho SY, McCarthy KP, Josen M, Rigby ML. Anatomic-echocardiographic correlates: an introduction to normal and congenitally malformed hearts. *Heart* 2001; **86**: ii3–11 (free PDF).

Ntsinjana HN, Hughes ML, Taylor AM.
The role of cardiovascular magnetic resonance in pediatric congenital heart disease. *J Cardiovasc Magn Reson* 2011; **13**: 51, available at www.jcmr-online.com/content/13/1/51.

Wang YC, Huang CH. Intraoperative transesophageal echocardiography for congenital heart disease, available at www.intechopen.com/download/pdf/26294.

Wilkinson JL. Haemodynamic calculations in the catheter laboratory. *Heart* 2001; **85**: 113–20 (free PDF).

4

Arterial Shunts and Pulmonary Artery Banding

David J. Barron

Introduction

There are a number of conditions or clinical situations in which it is not possible or safe to correct the circulation. These can be divided into two groups:

1. Anatomies in which biventricular repair is not possible. This includes a whole variety of conditions that can be summarized as 'functionally univentricular circulations'. To be born with a truly single ventricle is vanishingly rare, and most of these conditions have a small, underdeveloped or hypoplastic ventricle on either the right or left side. This mixed bag of anatomical variants accounts for 3 to 4 per cent of all congenital heart disease but for 15 per cent of all congenital cardiac surgeries (because they all generally need a series of staged procedures).

2. Anatomies in which biventricular repair will be possible at a later age but which present in a neonate or small infant with inadequate pulmonary blood supply (e.g. pulmonary atresia or severe tetralogy of Fallot).

Since the list of anatomical variants is virtually endless, each patient needs to be assessed on an individual basis, and the morphology and anatomical connections must be carefully analyzed with echocardiography and clinical assessment. The key to managing any neonate with a functionally univentricular circulation is to achieve a balanced circulation: i.e. unobstructed venous inflow into the heart, unobstructed systemic outflow and a balanced pulmonary blood flow. In terms of the latter, anatomies that have pulmonary atresia or severe pulmonary/subpulmonary stenosis will require some form of securing additional pulmonary blood flow (a shunt), whereas anatomies with too much pulmonary blood flow will require a limiting band on the pulmonary artery.

Arterial Shunts

Most cases can be stabilized with the use of prostaglandin E2 (Prostin) to establish ductal patency – and hence are referred to as 'duct-dependent circulations'. However, the ductal flow is not truly secure (completely dependent on intravenous Prostin and can still gradually close or vary despite this) and is uncontrolled and can lead to pulmonary over-circulation and heart failure. Thus the aim of initial palliation in these situations is to provide a secure and controlled pulmonary blood supply. The choice of technique is essentially guided by pulmonary vascular resistance: a neonate will have high pulmonary vascular resistance (PVR; close to systemic at birth and gradually falling over the first five to six months of life to normal values) and so requires a source of blood flow at relatively high pressure – an arterial shunt. The duct is usually ligated at the same procedure to avoid over-circulation and/or competitive flow with the shunt (but it can be left open, expecting it to close after the prostaglandin is stopped).

Blalock-Taussig Shunt. Described in the 1940s, before the era of cardiopulmonary bypass or prosthetic grafts, the classical Blalock-Taussig (BT) shunt involved sacrificing the subclavian artery and turning it down to connect it directly into the ipsilateral pulmonary artery. Sacrificing the artery in a neonate or young infant is a relatively safe procedure in that the collateral supply to the arm is very rich. The modern operation uses an interposition Gore-Tex graft between the subclavian (or innominate) artery and the pulmonary artery (the 'modified BT shunt'; Figure 4.1) – this avoids having to sacrifice the artery but also provides more controlled pulmonary blood flow, the Gore-Tex tube providing a fixed resistance in the circulation. The procedure was traditionally performed via a thoracotomy and can be performed on either the left or right side.

(a)

(b)

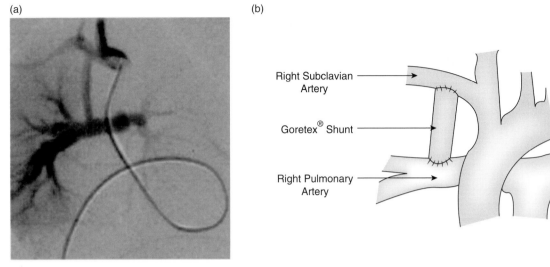

Right Subclavian Artery

Goretex® Shunt

Right Pulmonary Artery

Figure 4.1 Right modified Blalock-Taussig shunt. (A) Angiogram. The cardiac catheter is in the innominate artery and shows the shunt running between the subclavian artery and the right main pulmonary artery. (B) Diagram showing the anatomical position.

The right side is usually preferred as this allows the shunt to be taken from the distal innominate artery rather than the slightly smaller subclavian and also because the shunt will sit more medially (almost immediately behind the superior vena cava (SVC)), which makes it much easier to find and control at the subsequent procedure. If the aorta is a right arch, then the shunt is usually placed on the left side as the innominate artery is left sided.

The BT shunt is now more commonly performed via a median sternotomy. The advantages of this are mainly to avoid a thoracotomy scar for the child and easy access to the ductus to ligate it. The approach also allows for the ready use of cardiopulmonary bypass should the haemodynamics be unstable during the procedure. However, it is preferable to avoid bypass, if possible.

The choice of shunt size has evolved through trial and error over the years, and most neonates would receive a 3.5-mm shunt. A 3-mm shunt can be used for smaller neonates, and occasionally a 4-mm shunt is used in older neonates or for more distal shunts (such as those placed via thoracotomy).

In some anatomies, an alternative to the BT shunt can be to place a small (4–5 mm) right ventricle–to–pulmonary artery (RV-to-PA) conduit to provide pulmonary blood flow. This has the advantage of sustaining diastolic pressure (analogous to use of the RV-to-PA shunt in the Norwood operation; see Chapter 20), and in the setting of a biventricular anatomy such as

pulmonary atresia with VSD, it will also deliver predominantly desaturated blood into the lungs – rather than partially oxygenated blood as in the case of a BT shunt. This is only feasible in the right ventricle is of adequate size and has the disadvantage of requiring cardiopulmonary bypass and the need to create a ventriculotomy. Nevertheless, the more stable haemodynamics have given this approach increased popularity.

Central Shunt

An alternative method of delivering additional pulmonary blood flow is to construct a shunt directly from the aorta rather than from one of its branches. If the origin of the shunt is from the aorta, then it is referred to as a 'central shunt' (the term does not refer to a median sternotomy approach, since the shunt could be performed via sternotomy or thoracotomy). These shunts have the advantage of delivering higher flow and can be used if the head and neck artery anatomy is not suitable (e.g. no innominate artery or small vessels). Classically, central shunts were performed as direct anastomoses between the back of the ascending aorta and the right pulmonary artery (Waterston shunt; Figure 4.2) or between the front of the descending aorta and the left pulmonary artery (Potts shunt; Figure 4.3). These are now of historical interest only, although adult patients may still be encountered who had these procedures as children (meaning that the aorta and pulmonary artery will be fused together at these points). The current

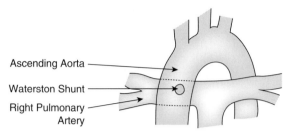

Figure 4.2 Waterston shunt. Direct communication is created between the back of the ascending aorta and the right pulmonary artery. This was an early form of 'central shunt' and is now generally performed by placing a small Gore-Tex shunt between the ascending aorta and the pulmonary artery.

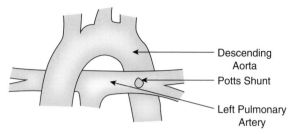

Figure 4.3 Potts shunt. This is created between the descending aorta and the posterior surface of the left pulmonary artery. It was performed through a left thoracotomy but has now been superseded by a small 'central shunts' of Gore-Tex placed between the aorta and the pulmonary artery.

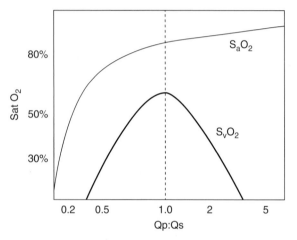

Figure 4.4 Relationship between arterial oxygen saturation (SaO_2) and mixed venous oxygen saturation (SvO_2) in the univentricular circulation with complete mixing of the pulmonary and systemic venous returns. The graphs show how the values change as the ratio of pulmonary-systemic blood flow (Qp:Qs) increases. Optimal conditions are achieved with maximum oxygen delivery (i.e. maximum SvO_2).

technique for central shunts is to use an interposition Gore-Tex graft from the ascending aorta to the most appropriate pulmonary artery. Again, these are ideally performed without cardiopulmonary bypass, although the need to place a side-biting clamp on the aorta may not be well tolerated and may require bypass support. As these shunts tend to be high flow and of shorter length, diameters are smaller than those chosen for a BT shunt, usually 3 or 3.5 mm.

Managing the Univentricular Circulation

There are two important guiding principles:

1. In all circulations that require a shunt, there will be a degree of obligate mixing of the 'blue' and 'red' bloodstreams. These are cyanotic heart conditions. The aim of postoperative management is to remember that there is only one source of flow (the systemic ventricle) for both pulmonary and systemic circulations. The aim is to achieve a pulmonary-to-systemic blood flow ratio Qp:Qs close to 1:1 – under-circulation to the lungs will result in hypoxia, but over-circulation will volume load the heart and potentially reduce systemic flow at the expense of the extra flow to the lungs – resulting in decreased oxygen delivery to the tissues despite a higher arterial partial pressure of oxygen (PO_2). This paradox is summarized in Figure 4.4, which shows that the minimum arteriovenous oxygen gap is achieved at a Qp:Qs of around 1:1. Assuming that mixed venous saturations are around 60 per cent, this equates to an arterial oxygen saturation (SaO_2) of around 80 per cent (presuming no parenchymal lung disease).

2. All arterial shunts will have continuous flow with a resultant decrease in diastolic systemic blood pressure and a wider pulse pressure.
   The consequence is a potential risk to coronary blood flow due to 'coronary steal' phenomenon during diastole. This can lead to sudden coronary ischaemia and haemodynamic collapse. Thus care has to be taken to avoid with pulmonary over-circulation and sudden falls in pulmonary vascular resistance, which can exacerbate the drop in diastolic pressure. Over-ventilation (dropping the partial pressure of carbon dioxide ($PaCO_2$)) or administration of high fraction of inspired oxygen (FiO_2) can precipitate such events and should be avoided. The underlying morphology must be born in mind when assessing each patient – for

example, a BT shunt in a Fallot will have an additional source of (systemic venous) pulmonary blood flow (through the native outflow tract) and so may generate slightly higher saturations without such risk of over-circulating.

The tendency in these circulations is towards pulmonary over-circulation, and early postoperative management is targeted at avoiding this – smaller shunts in the recent era have helped protect the situation, often accepting slightly lower PaO_2 in favour of better systemic perfusion. Systemic vasodilatation may help stabilize the circulation. Nevertheless, systemic shunts continue to carry a significant postoperative mortality in the modern era, reflecting the fragility of this circulation and the increasing complexity of the underlying conditions that are treated – 3 to 5 per cent mortality amongst neonates, with patient weight less than 3 kg remaining an important risk factor.

The Gore-Tex shunts are at risk of thrombosis, and patients are all given anti-platelet therapy of either aspirin or aspirin plus dipyrimadole. There is more recent interest in using more potent anti-platelet therapies such as clopidogrel, and all patients should be closely followed up for any early signs of shunt thrombosis or narrowing.

Pulmonary Artery Banding

Just as the arterial shunts provide a means of palliating the circulations with inadequate pulmonary blood flow, a pulmonary artery (PA) band is a means of palliating excessive pulmonary blood flow. The technique creates (supra-) pulmonary stenosis by placing a limiting circumferential band around the main pulmonary artery. This is a simple and effective way of reducing the Qp:Qs and so preventing over-circulation.

In its simplest setting, the PA band could be used in a baby with a large ventricular septal defect (VSD) to protect the lungs from high flows and pressures, the idea being to create a Fallot-type combination of VSD with pulmonary stenosis, which, we know, is a stable circulation. So long as the band is not made too tight, the baby will not become significantly cyanosed but remain well balanced.

Indications. A PA band can be used in any situation in which there is pulmonary over-circulation with consequent high-volume cardiac failure. However, as neonatal surgery has advanced, there has been a general trend towards early complete repair for the

majority of lesions. For example, in the early 1980s, a neonate with a large VSD may have been initially palliated with a PA band with the plan for subsequent VSD closure with de-banding when the child was older. In the modern day, the majority of neonatal VSDs would undergo primary closure. However, there are situations in the newborn in which a band is still more appropriate:

1. **Biventricular Circulations.** Multiple VSDs (classically, the 'Swiss cheese' multiple apical muscular VSDs which will naturally close over time, but the circulation needs balancing in the meantime), very small or premature babies (<2 kg), situations where bypass would be hazardous (e.g. intra-cerebral bleed, necrotizing enterocolitis).

2. **Functionally Univentricular Circulations.** Many patterns of functionally univentricular circulation may have unrestricted pulmonary blood flow – typically double-inlet left ventricle (DILV), tricuspid atresia with VSD or unbalanced atrio-ventricular septal defect (AVSD). It is essential that all aspects of the circulation are assessed independently. Frequently, other abnormalities such as hypoplastic aortic arch are present and must be addressed at the same time as banding The principle is always to ensure unobstructed inflow to the ventricular chamber, unobstructed systemic outflow and a balanced Qp:Qs.

A PA band also may be useful in situations of borderline sized left heart structures in the presence of a VSD. In this situation, the PA band is a safe option that allows the right ventricle (RV) to help support the systemic circulation if there is concern over the left ventricle (LV) size.

In the first group, there will be a degree of 'streaming' of the blood flow such that the majority of the systemic venous blood will still be directed to the lungs. Thus the oxygen saturations should still be well maintained in the nineties even with a relatively tight band. However, in functionally univentricular circulations, there will be a degree of obligate mixing of the bloodstreams at the atrial and ventricular levels, so the balanced circulation (in terms of Qp:Qs) will by necessity be at a lower arterial saturation, typically 80 to 85 per cent.

Procedure. Careful assessment of the anatomy by echocardiography is essential, particularly in uni-ventricular situations. Usually the band is placed via median sternotomy, and cardiopulmonary

(a)

(b)

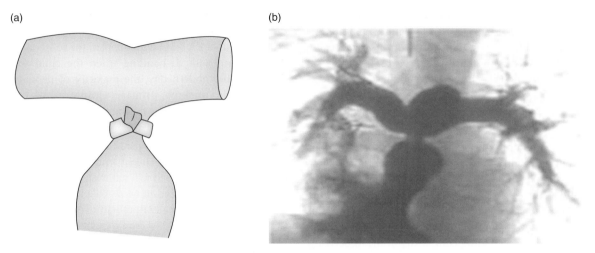

Figure 4.5 Pulmonary artery band. (A) Diagram showing the positioning of the band between the sino-tubular junction of the pulmonary valve and the bifurcation. Various materials can be used for the band, but most common is a 3-mm-diameter nylon tape or piece of Gore-Tex. (B) Angiogram showing band in place.

bypass will not be necessary unless other intracardiac procedures have to be addressed simultaneously. The pulmonary artery anatomy must be carefully defined such that the band can be placed safely in the correct position, immediately above the sino-tubular junction but not encroaching on the origins of the branch pulmonary arteries (Figure 4.5). The band material needs to be strong but atraumatic, typically a 3-mm-wide nylon tape or small strip of Gore-Tex. The key to the procedure is to achieve the correct tightness, which is a process of trial and error based on experience: it must be sufficient to generate adequate limitation of flow without being so tight that Qp:Qs is too limited. This can be done in a variety of ways, either by echocardiographic guidance based on the Doppler velocity across the band or by direct pressure measurement of the distal PA pressure, aiming to achieve one-half to one-third systemic pressures. An effective band should also generate an increase in systemic pressure due to better balancing of the circulation, and echocardiographic guidance will also ensure accurate positioning such that the band does not distort the pulmonary valve or the origins of the branch PAs. Trusler's law provides a good starting point for the surgeon, stating that the band circumference should be 20 mm plus 1 mm per kilogram body weight – minor adjustments can then be made using the techniques described earlier.

The band is fixed in place with a non-absorbable suture, and once the required circumference is chosen, it should also be fixed to the adventitia of the PA at a minimum of two points to prevent the band from migrating distally over time. Use of the SaO_2 can also be useful, but it must be remembered that this can vary according to the underlying anatomy and indication for the band: in a biventricular circulation, the saturations will be higher than in a mixing circulation, so again the pressure measurements and echocardiographic appearance are more useful than the SaO_2.

Occasionally, the band can be placed via a left thoracotomy, if preferred (especially if a coarctation is present that needs repairing), but it can be more difficult to place the band accurately and more difficult to assess on echocardiogram.

Further Reading

Brown S, Boshoff D, Rega F et al. Dilatable pulmonary artery banding in infants with low birth weight or complex congenital heart disease allows avoidance or postponement of subsequent surgery. *Eur J Cardiothorac Surg* 2010; **37**: 296–301.

Di Donato RM, Jonas RA, Lang P et al. Neonatal repair of tetralogy of Fallot with and without pulmonary atresia *J Thorac Cardiovasc Surg* 1991; **101**: 126–37.

Kolcz J, Pizarro C. Neonatal repair of tetralogy of Fallot results in improved pulmonary artery development without increased need for reintervention. *Eur J Cardiothorac Surg* 2005; **28**: 394–99.

Oka N, Brizard CP, Liava'a M, d'Udekem Y. Absorbable pulmonary arterial banding: an optimal strategy for muscular or residual ventricular septal defects. *J Thorac Cardiovasc Surg* 2011; **141**: 1081–82.

Petrucci O, O'Brien SM, Jacobs ML et al. Risk factors for mortality and morbidity after the neonatal Blalock-Taussig shunt procedure. *Ann Thorac Surg* 2011; **92**: 642–65.

Pigula FA, Khalil PN, Mayer JE, del Nido PJ, Jonas RA. Repair of tetralogy of Fallot in neonates and young infants. *Circulation* 1999; **100**: II157–61.

Trusler GA, Mustard WT. A method of banding the pulmonary artery for large isolated ventricular septal defect with and without transposition of the great arteries. *Ann Thorac Surg* 1972; **13**(4): 351–55.

Williams JA, Bansal AK, Kim BJ et al. Two thousand Blalock-Taussig shunts: a six-decade experience. *Ann Thorac Surg* 2007; **84**: 2070–75.

Yoshimura N, Yamaguchi M, Oka S, Yoshida M, Murakami H. Pulmonary artery banding still has an important role in the treatment of congenital heart disease. *Ann Thorac Surg* 2005; **79**: 1463.

Chapter 5

Patent Arterial Duct

Phil Botha

Introduction

The arterial duct originates from the sixth aortic arch and in fetal life allows the majority of fetal right ventricular output to be diverted away from the lungs to the lower body and placenta. The arterial duct is structurally composed of a thicker intima than adjacent vessels, prominent media with spirally arranged smooth muscle and an adventitia. During normal fetal development, the arterial ductal smooth muscle becomes increasingly sensitive to arterial oxygen tension such that the abrupt increase at birth causes constriction of the ductal smooth muscle. This effect is blunted by circulating prostaglandins, predominantly derived from the placenta. Following delivery, the level of placentally derived prostaglandin and prostacyclin falls precipitously, and metabolism by the lung increases. This renders the ductal smooth muscle more sensitive to oxygen, initiating a vasoconstriction response. Subsequent necrosis of the inner wall and fibrosis ultimately lead to complete obliteration of the duct. Ductal closure is complete within two weeks of birth in two-thirds of term patients and nearly all by one year of age. Persistent patency of the duct in a full-term infant is defined as patency beyond three months of age. This anomaly makes up 12 to 15 per cent of congenital heart defects and up to 30 per cent of defects found in premature infants. Eighty per cent of premature infants weighing less than 1,200 g will present with this condition.

Clinical Presentation

With increasing prematurity and lower birth weight, the immaturity of the ductal vasoconstrictor response results in an inability of the arterial duct to occlude post-natally. As the pulmonary vascular resistance falls, increasing left-to-right shunt will occur. The magnitude of the shunt will depend predominantly on the size of the patent ductus arteriosus (PDA), and the resultant runoff causes a low diastolic pressure and even reversal of flow in the descending aorta during diastole. This can cause reduced end-organ perfusion and an increased incidence of necrotizing enterocolitis, broncho-pulmonary dysplasia and cerebral bleeding complications. In older infants, the increased pulmonary blood flow can be entirely asymptomatic and is diagnosed after hearing a murmur or when it causes failure to thrive and recurrent chest infections. Large PDAs place a significant over-circulation and result in congestive cardiac failure and pulmonary hypertension if untreated.

In duct-dependent congenital cardiac lesions, part (or all) of the systemic circulation depends on the patency of the arterial duct for supply. Examples include aortic interruption and infantile coarctation of the aorta and various degrees of left heart hypoplasia. Similarly, any condition with pulmonary atresia or critical pulmonary stenosis depends on ductal patency to provide adequate pulmonary blood flow. In these conditions, maintaining or re-establishing ductal patency through infusion of synthetic prostaglandin E2 is lifesaving and allows for resuscitation and diagnostic workup before urgent repair is undertaken. In cyanotic heart conditions, prostaglandin infusion can also increase mixing at the ductal level to allow adequate saturations to be maintained until surgical repair is undertaken.

Clinical Findings and Management

Large PDAs will cause signs of congestive heart failure in neonates and infants with lung congestion, tachypnoea, poor feeding and enlarged liver edge. There is a 'machinery murmur' in both systole and diastole, heard loudest in the second intercostal space and radiating over the back. Pulses are usually bounding with wide pulse pressure. CXR shows enlarged heart with plethoric lungs, and the ECG may show some left ventricular hyperplasia (LVH) in older infants and children. Diagnosis is confirmed on echocardiography (Figure 5.1).

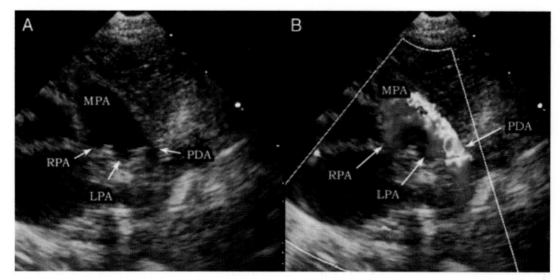

Figure 5.1 Echo images of a moderate-sized PDA and the trifurcating vies of the main and branch pulmonary arteries. (A black-and-white version of this figure will appear in some formats. For the colour version, please refer to the plate section.)

Despite the frequent occurrence of patent arterial duct and the seemingly simple nature of the defect, considerable controversy still exists regarding its management. Prior to widespread antibiotic therapy and surgical closure, infective endarteritis, ductal aneurysms and pulmonary vascular disease due to long-term left-to-right shunt were significant problems but are now seen rarely. No adequate randomized, placebo-controlled trial has been undertaken, and therefore, the timing and indications for closure of a PDA remain under debate. As safe options for trans-catheter occlusion of PDAs have become available, the vast majority of infants and children over 4 kg in weight will be treated by the percutaneous route, and surgical ligation in this group has become rare.

The majority of patients referred for PDA ligation in current practice are therefore very small, premature neonates, typically smaller than 1.5 kg. A trial of expectant management is indicated in all premature neonates without lung disease of prematurity (usually >1.5 kg in weight), as the majority of ducts will close spontaneously. If the duct is large and persistent and the neonate symptomatic (failing attempts to wean from ventilation) with signs of left heart volume overload on echocardiogram, most centres would advocate a course of medical management in the first instance. In borderline cases, the traditional echocardiographic criterion of a significant PDA was that the diameter of the

left atrium on a long-axis parasternal view was more than 1.5 times the diameter of the ascending aorta – indicating a large volume load on the left heart. However, the indication is usually more subjective, guided by a history of a premature neonate failing to wean from ventilation with clear evidence of a moderate or large PDA and pulmonary congestion on CXR.

Traditionally, this has comprised three doses of indomethacin, but recent randomized trials have demonstrated ibuprofen to have a lower incidence of intra-cerebral haemorrhage and renal dysfunction with similar efficacy. Some more recent randomized trials have found similar efficacy with paracetamol but with a lower incidence of renal impairment. If medical management has failed or is contra-indicated (such as the presence of an intra-cerebral bleed or necrotizing enterocolitis) and a haemodynamically significant PDA with left heart volume overload persists, PDA closure is indicated. Percutaneous device occlusion has been successful in children down to 1.2 kg in weight and can be undertaken through a 4F sheath inserted via the femoral artery in the majority of ductal anatomies (Figure 5.2). The most common complications reported are arterial injury and device embolization. In the presence of a very large duct, where device embolization poses a significant risk, and in very small babies, surgical duct ligation remains the therapeutic option of choice.

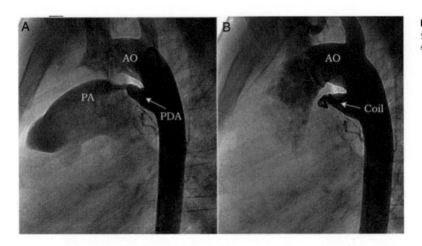

Figure 5.2 Angiographic images showing PDA occlusion with an endovascular coil.

Surgical Duct Ligation

The arterial duct is typically unilateral and ipsilateral to the side of the aortic arch. Rarely, bilateral arterial ducts can occur in pulmonary atresia and unusual forms of aortic interruption. Careful preoperative echocardiographic evaluation is mandatory to confirm the persistence of a significant arterial duct, exclude other major intra-cardiac abnormalities and confirm the side of the arch.

When a patent arterial duct exists in conjunction with significant intra-cardiac abnormality, duct ligation is typically undertaken during repair via median sternotomy. This is accomplished by dissection of the duct, taking care to avoid injury to the recurrent laryngeal nerve, and either suture ligation or application of a surgical clip. Adequate dissection to define pulmonary arterial and arch anatomy is mandatory to prevent inadvertent compromise of adjacent vessels.

In isolated PDA, ligation is performed via the left chest (in the usual setting of left aortic arch) using an open approach. A posterolateral muscle-sparing thoracotomy through the fourth intercostal space has been used in the majority of very small neonates and has proven safe and effective. Great care is taken to avoid injury to the visceral pleura during entry and lung retraction to avoid the risks of air leak and chest drainage in babies possibly requiring long-term ventilatory support. A thoracoscopic approach can be used and had been described in babies as small as 575 g but is generally only used in babies weighing more than 3 kg and is contra-indicated in cases of severe pulmonary dysfunction and possibly cases with a very large PDA. Since almost all surgical PDA closures are in neonates weighing less than 1.5 kg, the opportunities for thoracoscopic closure are very limited.

The anatomy and two described anatomical pitfalls are demonstrated in Figure 5.3. With the lung retracted medially, the parietal pleura is divided overlying the duct, and the PDA and aortic arch are dissected sufficiently to confirm the arch anatomy. The vagus and recurrent laryngeal nerves are carefully preserved by limiting dissection to the area immediately adjacent to the aorta. The duct is ligated using a braided ligature or a surgical clip is applied. Routine closure is undertaken, usually without a pleural drain. A pulse oximeter should always be placed on the lower limb to guard against inadvertent ligation of the aorta (due to the transverse arch being mistaken for the duct).

Outcomes. It is generally a very safe procedure, and any complications are usually related to the co-morbidities of severe prematurity. Bleeding due to the fragility of the duct can be life threatening, but the operative mortality is less than 1 per cent. Complications include left recurrent laryngeal nerve injury, chylous leak (rare) and pneumothorax due to inadvertent lung injury. Despite a low procedural risk, the 30-day mortality for the procedure is 5 to 10 per cent, reflecting the significant co-morbidities of these very premature neonates. Concern regarding long-term sequelae of thoracotomy, notably scoliosis, and failure to demonstrate improvement in outcomes after surgical duct ligation has prompted a less aggressive management strategy in very premature neonates by some. Only two small studies with relatively short follow-up have investigated this outcome, demonstrating a very low incidence of scoliosis.

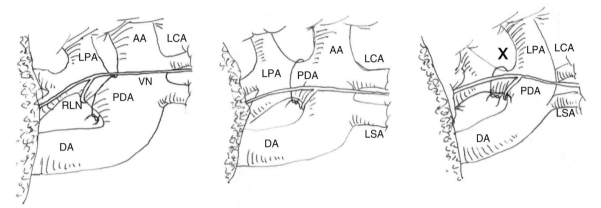

Figure 5.3 (a) Normal ductal anatomy as seen from the surgeon's perspective at left thoracotomy. Recurrent laryngeal nerve passes under the PDA. (B) Rare anatomical variant in which the PDA arises from the arch proximal to the left subclavian artery, and the right laryngeal nerve passes underneath the aortic arch. (C) Large PDA sweeping into the descending aorta appears to be the aortic arch. The aortic arch is obscured from view by the PDA, which can lead to inadvertent ligation of the left pulmonary artery. (AA = aortic arch; DA = descending aorta; LSA = left subclavian artery; LCA = left carotid artery; PDA = patent ductus arteriosus (arterial duct); LPA = left pulmonary artery; VN = vagus nerve; RLN = recurrent laryngeal nerve.
Source: Adapted from Pontius et al. Illusions leading to surgical closure of the distal left pulmonary artery instead of the ductus arteriosus. *J Thorac Cardiovasc Surg* 1981; 82(1): 107–13.

Further Reading

Mitra S, Rønnestad A, Holmstrøm H. Management of patent ductus arteriosus in preterm infants: where do we stand? *Congenital Heart Dis* 2013; **8**(6): 500–12.

Pontius RG, Danielson GK, Noonan JA, Judson JP. Illusions leading to surgical closure of the distal left pulmonary artery instead of the ductus arteriosus. *J Thorac Cardiovasc Surg* 1981; **82**(1): 107–13.

Stankowski T, Aboul-Hassan SS, Marczak J, Cichon R. Is thoracoscopic patent ductus arteriosus closure superior to conventional surgery? *Interact Cardiovasc Thorac Surg* 2015; **21**(4): 532–38.

Van Overmeire B, Smets K, Lecoutere D et al. A comparison of ibuprofen and indomethacin for closure of patent ductus arteriosus. *N Engl J Med* 2000; **343**(10): 674–81.

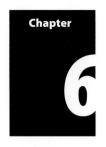

Coarctation of the Aorta and Aortic Interruption

Natasha Khan

Introduction

Coarctation of the aorta is defined as a congenital narrowing of the upper descending aorta/distal aortic arch opposite the arterial duct. This accounts for 5 to 8 per cent of all congenital heart defects. It is an isolated finding in 25 per cent of cases but is associated with other cardiac lesions in 75 per cent, most commonly ventricular septal defect (VSD). There is a strong association with bicuspid aortic valve (25–40 per cent). It is the most common cardiac defect in Turner syndrome.

Morphology and Histology

The constriction consists of localized medial thickening with infolding of medial and neointimal layers. It may form a shelf within the lumen of the aorta or may be concentric narrowing. The constriction may be discrete or, more rarely, a long tubular segment. All congenital coarctations are related to the site of duct insertion ('juxtaductal') with a 'ductal sling' of tissue encircling the aorta; however, coarctations that are inflammatory or autoimmune in aetiology may develop in the descending thoracic aorta or abdominal aorta, although they are extremely rare. There is commonly a degree of hypoplasia of the isthmus of the aorta, just proximal to the coarctation, and the transverse arch may be hypoplastic. Untreated coarctation can develop significant collateral vessels from proximal to the coarctation to the lower part of the body.

Coarctation may be a feature of more complex cardiac defects, typically those with a left-right shunt, such as VSD, atrio-ventricular septal defect (AVSD) transposition of the great arteries (TGA)/VSD and Taussig-Bing syndrome. It is also commonly seen as part of hypoplastic left heart syndrome, where there tends to be more extensive arch hypoplasia, and also as part of the constellation of left-sided obstructive lesions known as the 'Shone complex'.

Pathophysiology and Natural History

The severity of the coarctation dictates the age of presentation. Severe cases present in neonates, usually as the ductus closes in the first few days of life. The haemodynamic consequences are a rapidly increasing afterload on the left ventricle leading to acute left ventricular failure and under-perfusion of the body beyond the coarctation and circulatory collapse.

In less severe coarctation, left ventricular (LV) failure is less likely, but LV hypertrophy and systemic hypertension gradually evolve. There is development of collateral circulation bypassing the coarcted segment. In infancy, congestive heart failure rarely occurs, and these children are usually asymptomatic and diagnosed only on chance clinical findings. Hypertension develops due to the mechanical obstruction and the activation of renin-angiotensin-mediated pathways.

Uncorrected coarctation leads to a curtailed life expectancy of 30 to 40 years, with causes of death including aortic rupture, intra-cranial haemorrhage, cardiac failure, accelerated coronary artery disease and bacterial endocarditis. Beyond infancy, even after correction, there is a lifetime risk of hypertension and its sequelae. After correction, freedom from complications or hypertension is only 20 per cent at 25 years.

Presentation

Neonates present with collapse, acidosis, hypotension, heart failure and absent femoral pulses. During infancy, there may be a degree of congestive heart failure causing dyspnoea and failure to thrive; femoral pulses may be weak.

Children/Young Adults. Most commonly diagnosed on chance finding of abnormal CXR, ECG or hypertension. May present with headaches, lower extremity weakness, exertional dyspnoea and, rarely, stroke or a transient ischaemic attack (TIA). Examination reveals radio-femoral delay or weak femoral pulses, with differential blood pressure between upper and lower limbs.

CXR may show the classic '3', or hourglass, sign of a coarctation along the contour of the upper mediastinum and rib notching on the underside of the ribs (caused by the large intercostal collateral vessels) The heart shadow may be enlarged if there is a degree of heart failure. The ECG shows left ventricular hypertrophy (LVH).

Echocardiography. In neonates, infants and young children, trans-thoracic echo is diagnostic. Doppler measures the velocity across the coarctation, enabling estimation of the pressure gradient. Colour flow mapping demonstrates the diastolic 'tail' of persistently raised velocity in the descending aorta. The aortic valve should be carefully assessed to examine for bicuspid morphology.

In older children and young adults, MRI or CT scan becomes the imaging modality of choice, giving excellent delineation of the aortic anatomy and extent and size of collateral vessels. These modalities are not usually necessary in younger children if echo has provided clear definition of the anatomy.

Management of the Collapsed Neonate

Neonates may require resuscitation with intubation, ventilation and inotropic support if necessary. Prostaglandin E2 is essential to attempt to reopen the duct (usually successful because the duct has only just closed) and will usually stabilize the circulation. Surgery usually can be delayed until the patient is stable but is generally performed within the next 24 hours.

In an older child, hypertension should be treated, usually with beta-blockers, but surgery should not be delayed while waiting for normotension.

Surgery

Choice of technique and surgical approach depends on the age of the patient, the extent of the lesion and the presence of any associated cardiac defects. Neonates and infants with isolated coarctation are treated in one of two ways, usually via left posterolateral thoracotomy.

Resection and Extended End-to-End Anastomosis. The site of the coarctation, the descending aorta, and the arch as far forward as the ascending aorta can all be mobilized and controlled. Clamps are placed on the descending aorta and on the arch as far forward as the left carotid artery. The coarctation segment and the isthmus are resected. The opening into the distal arch is extended forwards, and the two open ends are then anastomosed together (Figure 6.1). In extreme cases, the isthmus can be ligated and an incision made more anteriorly into the underside of the arch – the descending aorta is then brought up into this opening (an 'end-to-side' anastomosis). Care must be taken not to create too much tension in the arch, which can trap the left main bronchus.

Subclavian Flap Angioplasty. (Figure 6.2) The aorta is mobilized and clamps placed across the descending aorta and transverse arch. The left subclavian artery is ligated distally, transected and then laid open along its length, extending the incision across the site of the coarctation. The opened subclavian artery is then folded down and used as a flap to enlarge the narrowed segment. This technique has the disadvantage of leaving the coarctation ridge in situ, which can lead to a higher recurrence rate and sacrifices the subclavian artery (which is well tolerated in neonates but can lead to slight hemi-smallness of the left arm).

In older infants and children, balloon angioplasty is the first choice for localized coarctation, but if ballooning is unsuccessful or if there is associated

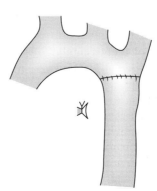

Figure 6.1 Coarctation repair with resection and extended end-to-end anastomosis. The dotted lines show the points at which the aorta is transected. The arrow shows the extended incision made into the underside of the arch to widen the proximal anastomosis.

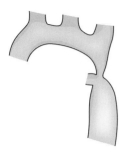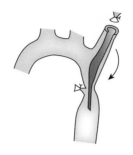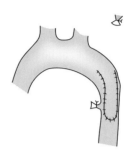

Figure 6.2 Coarctation repair using subclavian flap technique. The left subclavian artery is ligated and divided distally. The artery is then laid open, extending this incision across the site of coarctation, and then turned down to augment the narrowed segment.

arch hypoplasia, then surgery may be required. Direct anastomosis remains the technique of choice but becomes more difficult in older children, in whom the vessels are less elastic. In older children, an interposition graft can be placed as long as an adult-sized graft can be accommodated, but this is becoming increasingly rare as balloon angioplasty and the use of intravascular stents become more feasible.

Children of any age with associated arch hypoplasia may be best treated via median sternotomy, mobilizing the arch and descending aorta on bypass. The coarctation segment is resected and the transverse arch laid open, coming as anteriorly as necessary. The posterior wall of the aorta is reconstructed end to end, and the opening in the concavity of the arch is then augmented with a patch (typically pulmonary homograft or xenograft pericardium). This is a reliable technique and is ideal if there are concomitant intra-cardiac lesions that require attention (e.g. VSD).

An alternative approach for discrete coarctation with VSD is to repair the aorta via a left thoracotomy and place a pulmonary artery band. However, there is an increasing trend towards single-stage repair for combined lesions such as these, repairing both the arch and VSD via median sternotomy on bypass.

Simple patch repair of the coarctation segment in older children is generally not recommended due to the high incidence of recurrent coarctation and of late false aneurysm at the suture lines. Adults presenting with re-coarctation usually can be successfully treated with balloon angioplasty and stent placement. If stenting is not feasible, or if there is associated transverse arch hypoplasia, then surgery can be considered – using an interposition graft via sternotomy or left thoracotomy with left heart bypass. Extra-anatomic grafts from the ascending aorta to the descending aorta (approached through the posterior

pericardium) can avoid having to access the site of complex re-coarctation.

Outcome. Isolated coarctation carries a perioperative risk of death of 1 to 2 per cent. Early complications include a 0.4 per cent risk of paraplegia (associated with long cross-clamp times and division of collaterals) and damage to the recurrent laryngeal nerve or the thoracic duct. The incidence of chylothorax is less than 3 per cent in neonates/infants but slightly higher in older patients. Transient renal failure and necrotizing enterocolitis may occur, particularly in collapsed neonates with poor distal perfusion preoperatively.

Late complications are of recurrent coarctation (>85 per cent successfully treated with catheter intervention) and persistent hypertension. The risk of hypertension is much less if the patient is repaired at less than 5 years of age, but in older patients, up to 50 per cent may still have hypertension requiring medical therapy. Late false aneurysm can occur at the suture lines of patch repairs or interposition grafts, and these patients should have life-long follow-up to screen for these problems.

Aortic Interruption

This is defined as an interruption of luminal continuity between the ascending and descending aorta. The arch is usually two completely separate components rather than fibrous atresia. It is rare, comprising less than 1 per cent of congenital cardiac defects.

Morphology

There are three possible points of interruption, correlating with the different embryonic derivations of the aortic arch:

- **Type A interruption** (25–35 per cent). At the isthmus, just distal to the left subclavian artery (LSCA) origin

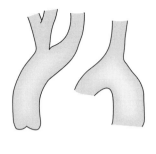

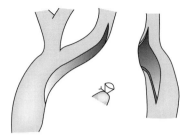

Figure 6.3 Interrupted arch type B. Technique of repair with direct anastomosis and patch augmentation.

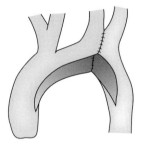

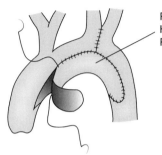

Pulmonary Homograft Patch

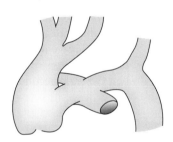

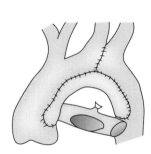

Figure 6.4 Aortic interruption type B with truncus arteriosus. The same technique of interruption repair can be used, with direct anastomosis and patch augmentation.

- **Type B** (60–70 per cent). Between the left coronary cusp (LCC) and the LSCA, often associated with aberrant RSCA and sub-aortic stenosis
- **Type C** (5 per cent). Between the innominate and LCC arteries

Interrupted arch is almost always associated with a left-to-right intra-cardiac shunt: VSD 80 to 90 per cent, common arterial trunk 10 per cent and aorto-pulmonary window in 5 to 10 per cent. It is also associated with bicuspid aortic valve in 60 per cent, sub-aortic stenosis in 20 per cent and Di George syndrome in 33 to 50 per cent.

Pathophysiology and Natural History

The patent arterial duct is the only source of blood supply distal to the interruption. Ductal closure leads to a sudden decrease in blood flow to the trunk and lower body, causing systemic hypoperfusion, acidosis, renal failure, necrotizing enterocolitis and hepatic ischaemia. Neonates present when the duct closes, with circulatory shock and congestive cardiac failure. They must be resuscitated, with a prostaglandin infusion, inotropes, if necessary, and intubation and ventilation to allow easy manipulation of the pulmonary vascular bed and thus ductal flow.

There may be abnormal pulse patterns depending on the site of interruption. Even if the duct remains open, neonates may present with cardiac failure related to the associated lesions (large VSD or truncus arteriosus).

CXR shows cardiomegaly and pulmonary vascular congestion; the aortic knuckle is absent. ECG shows right ventricular hypertrophy

Echocardiography. Trans-thoracic echo is diagnostic, showing interruption of the aorta arch, descending aorta continuing from the duct. The head and neck vessels can be carefully delineated with a CT scan, which is useful if there is doubt about the pattern of interruption. Echo is important in defining the other cardiac anomalies that present in the majority of patients with interrupted arch.

Surgery

Surgical correction is indicated in all cases and may be by a staged correction or single-stage complete repair depending on the associated defects.

Arch Repair

The arch is repaired via a median sternotomy on cardiopulmonary bypass. (Occasionally, repair has been described through a thoracotomy; the descending aorta can be anastomosed end to side into the ascending aorta for short-segment interruption with good-sized arch components.)

Cardiopulmonary bypass is established with two arterial cannulae, one to the ascending aorta (often via a shunt placed into the innominate artery to allow better access to the ascending aorta for repair) and the other to the arterial duct, with a snare around the ductal cannula to occlude ductal flow on bypass. The patient is cooled to 18°C, with at least 20 minutes of cooling to achieve uniform temperatures. The heart is arrested, under deep hypothermic arrest. Using a combination of deep hypothermic circulatory arrest (DHCA) and anterograde cerebral perfusion, the arch of the aorta can be excluded from the circulation in order to perform the repair. The head and neck vessels are occluded, and the descending aorta is isolated in a clamp. All ductal tissue can now be excised from the aorta. An incision is made into the facing aspect of the proximal aorta, extending the incision up into the LSCA or LCC to enlarge the anastomosis. The back wall of the distal aorta is now anastomosed to the back wall of this proximal incision to restore continuity in the arch. There is not usually adequate tissue to perform a complete end-to-end anastomosis without tension, so the repair is usually augmented with a patch into the inner curvature of the arch using a pulmonary artery homograft patch, if available, or glutaraldehyde-treated pericardium, if not (Figure 6.3). If there is an aberrant RSCA arising from the descending thoracic aorta, it may impede full mobility of the aorta and may have to be sacrificed.

Other methods of repairing the arch include a 'sliding angioplasty' with the descending aorta brought up to anastomose end to side with the ascending aorta, using the SCA or carotid artery 'turned down' to augment the anastomosis or an interposition graft.

Single-Stage Complete Repair

The commonest presentation of interrupted arch with VSD is most commonly repaired completely in the neonatal period. This approach can also be used for interrupted arch in conjunction with anomalous pulmonary artery, anteroposterior window, common arterial trunk, total anomalous pulmonary venous connection (TAPVC), TGA, or Taussig-Bing syndrome.

Staged Repair

This will depend on the preoperative condition of the neonate and the nature of the associated lesions. In the setting of a large VSD, the arch may be repaired and the main pulmonary artery (PA) banded to prevent pulmonary overflow – with a plan for de-banding and VSD closure in the future. This is a pragmatic option for high-risk patients with complex anatomy or in whom there is doubt about the ability to achieve a two-ventricle circulation. The second stage of surgery, whether corrective or palliative, takes place when the child is bigger and when the band becomes too tight, causing desaturation.

Early Postoperative Care and Complications

The chest may be left open for the first 24 to 48 hours to stabilize haemodynamics. There is often a systemic inflammatory reaction and low cardiac output syndrome requiring inotropic support and occasionally peritoneal dialysis. There is evidence of left recurrent laryngeal nerve palsy in up to 40 per cent of patients, with the sequelae of requirement of non-invasive respiratory support and nasogastric (NG) feeding. Undue tension in the repair can lead to compression of the left main bronchus resulting in persistent collapse or air trapping of the left lung, compromising weaning from ventilatory support. Recurrent stenosis in the repaired arch is seen in 10 to 30 per cent of cases, although the majority are successfully treated with balloon dilatation.

Outcomes

Mortality for the single-stage repair is currently 10 to 20 per cent depending on the associated lesions. The risk of reoperation is no higher than with staged repair. The five-year survival is 65 to 70 per cent; late survival is less for those with left ventricular outflow tract obstruction (LVOTO). Ten-year freedom from all reoperation is 50 per cent, but freedom from reoperation on the arch is 85 to 90 per cent. The mortality for repair through a thoracotomy with PA banding is low, but long-term reinterventions are similar, and these are usually selected cases with favourable anatomy. A major risk factor for early and late mortality is low weight at surgery, with 10-year survival of 30 to 40 per cent in those operated on weighing less than 2.5 kg.

Further Reading

Barreiro CJ, Ellison TA, Williams JA et al. Subclavian flap aortoplasty: still a safe, reproducible, and effective treatment for infant coarctation. *Eur J Cardiothorac Surg* 2007; **31**(4): 649–53. Epub 2007.

Brown JW, Ruzmetov M, Okada Y et al. Outcomes in patients with interrupted aortic arch and associated anomalies: a 20-year experience. *Eur J Cardiothorac Surg* 2006; **29**(5): 666–73.

Brown ML, Burkhart HM, Connolly HM et al. Coarctation of the aorta: lifelong surveillance is mandatory following surgical repair. *J Am Coll Cardiol* 2013; **62**(11):1020–25.

Früh S, Knirsch W, Dodge-Khatami A et al. Comparison of surgical and interventional therapy of native and recurrent aortic coarctation regarding different age groups during childhood. *Eur J Cardiothorac Surg* 2011; **39**(6): 898–904.

Gaynor JW, Wernovsky G, Rychik J et al. Outcome following single-stage repair of coarctation with ventricular septal defect. *Eur J Cardiothorac Surg* 2000; **18**(1): 62–67.

Kaushal S, Backer CL, Patel JN et al. Coarctation of the aorta: midterm outcomes of resection with extended end-to-end anastomosis. *Ann Thorac Surg* 2009; **88**(6): 1932–38.

Lee MG, Brink J, Galati JC et al. End-to-side repair for aortic arch lesions offers excellent chances to reach adulthood without reoperation. Ann Thorac Surg 2014; **98** (4): 1405–11.

McCrindle BW, Tchervenkov CI, Konstantinov IE et al. Risk factors associated with mortality and interventions in 472 neonates with interrupted aortic arch: a Congenital Heart Surgeons Society study. *J Thorac Cardiovasc Surg* 2005; **129**: 343–50.

Mishra PK. Management strategies for interrupted aortic arch with associated anomalies. *Eur J Cardiothorac Surg* 2009; **35**(4): 569–76.

Rajasinghe HA, Reddy VM, van Son JA et al. Coarctation repair using end-to-side anastomosis of descending aorta to proximal aortic arch. *Ann Thorac Surg* 1996; **61**(3): 840–44.

Sakurai T, Stickley J, Stümper O et al. Repair of isolated aortic coarctation over two decades: impact of surgical approach and associated arch hypoplasia. *Interact Cardiovasc Thorac Surg* 2012; **15**(5): 865–70.

Ungerleider RM, Pasquali SK, Welke KF et al. Contemporary patterns of surgery and outcomes for aortic coarctation: an analysis of the Society of Thoracic Surgeons Congenital Heart Surgery Database. *J Thorac Cardiovasc Surg* 2013; **145**(1): 150–57.

Walters HL 3rd, Ionan CE, Thomas RL, Delius RE. Single-stage versus two-stage repair of coarctation of the aorta with ventricular septal defect. *J Thorac Cardiovasc Surg* 2008; **135** (4): 754–61.

Atrial Septal Defects

Natasha Khan

Introduction

Atrial septal defects (ASDs) defect in the atrial septum that lead to shunting of blood between left and right atria. They constitute 10 to 15 per cent of congenital cardiac defects and up to 40 per cent of congenital defects presenting in adulthood. Over 80 per cent of defects are secundum ASDs or stretched patent foramen ovale (PFO).

The atrial septum is made up mainly of the flap valve of the oval fossa surrounded by the thickened superior rim or 'limbus' superiorly and laterally. This is the 'true' atrial septum, as the remainder of the 'septum secundum' is actually infolded atrial wall rather than septal structures. The foramen ovale lies at the superior end of the oval fossa and usually closes as the pressures in the atria reverse after birth (see Chapter 1), closing the flap valve against the limbus. Persistence of this hole, in the form of a PFO represents the commonest form of interatrial communication.

Types of ASD

Patent foramen ovale (PFO). The oval fossa may be probe patent in 25 to 30 per cent of humans, detectable in up to 15 to 20 per cent of adults with echocardiography. The PFO can become stretched such that it becomes a significant opening located superiorly in the fossa ovalis. Large defects become indistinguishable from a secundum ASD.

Secundum ASD. This involves defects of the true atrial septum, the septum secundum. There is complete or partial absence of the floor of the oval fossa, and there may be remnant strands of septal tissue that create the appearance of fenestrations or of multiple neighbouring defects. Frequently these defects extend close to the inferior vena cava (IVC) opening.

Sinus Venosus ASD. This is an interatrial communication (10 per cent) related to the point where the

superior vena cava (SVC) or the IVC enters the atrium (these defects can also be described as 'the caval vein having a biatrial connection'). The majority are superior sinus venosus ASDs, at the mouth of the SVC, which is associated in 90 per cent of cases with an anomalous right upper pulmonary vein from the upper and/or middle lobe draining into this junction.

Primum ASDs. Also called 'partial atrio-ventricular septal defects', these defects constitute an absence of the primum atrial septum. The defect is crescentic in shape, and the medial margin is the valve leaflets of the atrio-ventricular (A-V) valves – thus there is no atrial tissue between the defect and the valve leaflets. These defects are part of the spectrum of atrio-ventricular septal defects and are dealt with in detail in Chapter 10.

Coronary Sinus ASD. These are varying communications between the coronary sinus and the left atrium (<3 per cent), also known as 'unroofed coronary sinus'. When the coronary sinus is completely unroofed, the orifice of the coronary sinus is essentially an opening into the left atrium – hence an ASD. This defect can be associated with persistent left SVC (see Figure 7.1).

Pathophysiology and Natural History

ASDs permit left-to-right shunting, causing volume overload of the right heart and increased pulmonary blood flow. The magnitude and direction of flow through any ASD depend on the size of the ASD and the relative diastolic filling properties/compliance of the left and right ventricles.

The shunt in isolated ASD is left to right. A significant shunt is defined as one that has a pulmonary-to-systemic blood flow ratio Qp:Qs greater than 1.5:1 or is any shunt causing significant right heart dilatation. This chronic volume overload of the right heart causes pulmonary congestion which

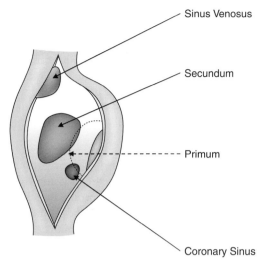

Figure 7.1 View through the right atrium showing the positions of atrial septal defects.

can predispose to recurrent chest infection, but haemodynamic symptoms are due to gradual right ventricular failure causing effort intolerance (not usually until the fourth or fifth decade). This can be worsened by the development of functional tricuspid incompetence and/or atrial fibrillation/flutter secondary to the chronic volume overload of the right heart. The high pulmonary blood flow associated with significant ASD is at low pressure and generally does *not* tend to precipitate increased pulmonary vascular resistance. Nevertheless, there is a small group of patients with ASDs (5 per cent of adults with untreated large ASDs) who will develop pulmonary hypertension if the ASD is not treated, although debate continues as to whether this is a manifestation of primary pulmonary hypertension rather than the ASD being the cause.

In patients operated on before age 25, right ventricle (RV) size and function would be expected to return to normal and life expectancy return to that of the normal population, However, repair at >25 years, although still conveying both symptomatic improvement and improved life expectancy, does not restore to normality. When ASDs are closed in childhood, the long-term risk of arrhythmias is not much higher than that of the general population, but after age 11, this risk increases so that about 50 per cent of 60-year-olds with ASD have atrial flutter or fibrillation or sinus node dysfunction.

ASDs rarely cause symptoms in children and are usually found incidentally or through investigations for recurrent chest infections. Rarely, if the defect is very big, there may be heart failure and failure to thrive (1 per cent of patients). If an infant or small child presents with heart failure, other associated lesions must be excluded, e.g. patent arterial duct or lesions causing high left atrial pressure. In older children and adolescents, there may be reduced exercise tolerance in comparison to peers. In older adults, presentation may be at the onset of atrial arrhythmias. Congestive heart failure may occurs in up to a third of patients over age 40.

Investigation

CXR shows pulmonary plethora with prominent hilar vessels and enlarged right heart. ECG can be normal in children but can show peaked P waves in II, V2 due to atrial enlargement, right-axis deviation (+100 degrees) and right ventricular strain pattern due to volume overload (RSR′ pattern V3, V1). In adults, atrial flutter/fibrillation may be seen and right bundle branch block (RBBB) may be present in more than 50 per cent of patients over age 60.

Echocardiography is the definitive investigation, and trans-thoracic echo is diagnostic in the vast majority of cases. Trans-oesophageal echo (TOE) is occasionally necessary, particularly in adults in whom trans-thoracic views are poor or in sinus venosus defects to confirm pulmonary venous drainage. Bubble contrast echocardiography is rarely necessary but can be helpful in smaller defects to prove an atrial shunt. Sinus venosus ASDs may be difficult to visualize, especially inferior sinus venosus defects, but can be better seen on TOE. MRI and CT scan are not routinely required.

Cardiac catheterization is rarely necessary unless there are concerns about pulmonary hypertension – to measure pulmonary vascular resistance and its reversibility with vasodilators. It is the most precise method to quantify the shunt (i.e. calculate Qp:Qs), but in practice, it is rarely necessary to calculate Qp:Qs unless there is genuine debate over whether a defect merits closure. The hallmark of an ASD is an increase in O_2 saturations of more than 5 per cent from the SVC to the right atrium.

Device Closure

A multitude of trans-catheter devices have been developed for ASD closure, and the technique has revolutionized management over the last 20 years such that it is now the treatment of choice for appropriate lesions. However, devices are *only* suitable for secundum ASDs or PFOs and *only* where there are adequate margins to accommodate the device.

The procedure is performed in the cardiac catheter laboratory. The device is placed across the atrial septum via a catheter in the femoral vein, with TOE guidance.

Complications include incomplete defect closure, device migration/erosion, and local vascular complications. Device migration/erosion may occur late, so long-term follow-up is required.

Surgery

All significant defects not suitable for device closure are referred for surgical closure (Table 7.1). Standard cardiopulmonary bypass techniques are used with bicaval cannulation and cardioplegic arrest performed at moderate hypothermia or at normothermia for simple defects such as secundum ASD. Although median sternotomy is the standard approach, a number of more cosmetically attractive alternatives have been used for simple defects – as listed in Table 7.2.

Secundum ASD. The right atrium is opened through an incision starting at the base of the right appendage running parallel to the A-V groove. The anatomy should be confirmed (PAPVD can be missed on echo) and the defect closed, usually using a patch of either autologous pericardium, xenograft pericardium or Gore-Tex according to personal preference. Moderate-sized defects, particularly stretched PFOs, can sometimes be closed by direct suture, but since most moderate-sized defects are closed with a device, most that come to surgery require patch repair. Care should be taken to confirm the position of the IVC because in large defects with no inferior rim, the Eustachian valve can be mistaken for the inferior margin of the defect so that patch closure ends up with committing the IVC to the left atrium. The left heart should be thoroughly de-aired before tying down the patch.

Sinus Venosus ASD. The anatomy of the right pulmonary veins and their relation to the SVC and right atrium (RA) must be determined by careful mobilization of these structures. The SVC must be cannulated high-up to provide adequate access (separately snaring the azygous vein if necessary). The atrium is opened with a high lateral incision so that it can be extended up into the root of the SVC if necessary (staying laterally to avoid the sinoatrial (SA) node). The defect is closed with a patch such that the pulmonary veins are committed through to the left atrium. If the anomalous veins enter high up, then it may be necessary to extend the incision up into the root of the SVC to gain better access. In this situation, there is a risk that the patch will partially obstruct SVC inflow. There are three ways to avoid such a SVC obstruction:

1. **Two-Patch Technique.** The atrial-SVC incision is closed with a separate diamond-shaped patch. This gives more volume to the SVC to accommodate flow.
2. **V-Y Plasty.** An inverted Y-shaped incision is made in the atrium up into the root of the SVC. It is then closed as a V shape to widen the SVC root.

Table 7.1 Indications for Closure of an Atrial Septal Defect

Qp:Qs > 1.5
Any ASD with evidence of volume loading of the RV and accompanying symptoms
Infants with large ASD, failure to thrive, and/or recurrent lower respiratory tract infection (LRTI)
Any ASD with proven history of embolic stroke or transient ischaemic attack (TIA)
Sinus venosus defects with associated partial anomalous pulmonary venous drainage (PAPVD)
Coronary sinus defects with left SVC (obligate right-to-left shunt)
In adults with raised pulmonary vascular resistance (PVR), closure should be performed if Qp:Qs > 1.5 and PVR < 10 Wood units

Table 7.2 Alternative Surgical Approach for Secundum ASD

Right anterior thoracotomy – standard bypass cannulation
Right anterior thoracotomy – minimal-access cannulation
Right axillary, lateral or posterolateral approaches
Subxiphoid incision – with retraction of the sternum
Submammary Incision – bilateral submammary transverse incision with mobilization of soft tissues and median sternotomy
Robotic repair – minimal-access cannulation and thoracoscopic instrumentation

3. **Warden Procedure.** If a pulmonary vein drains very high, then the SVC can be transected just above this point. The ASD is then closed, committing the whole SVC root through to the left atrium, and the transected SVC is either over-sewn or closed with a patch. An opening is then made into the apex of the right atrial appendage, and the distal SVC is now anastomosed into this opening, restoring normal systemic venous return. Care must be taken not to purse-string this anastomosis, narrowing the SVC.

An alternative approach gaining some popularity is the trans-caval approach using a vertical incision in the SVC, never crossing the cavo-atrial junction, and using a patch to redirect anomalous pulmonary veins via the ASD into the left atrium (LA).

Inferior sinus venosus defects are extremely rare. Again, the pulmonary veins must be inspected carefully and the patch placed to commit them through to the LA. Since the IVC is usually a large opening, there is less risk of narrowing the inflow – if necessary, the inferior caval cannula is removed to expose this area better.

Coronary Sinus ASD. The repair of unroofed coronary sinus (CS) is simple in the absence of a persistent left SVC – the atrial defect created by the opening of the coronary sinus is simply closed with a patch, committing the CS to the LA (the coronary venous return thus creates a small right-to-left shunt, but this is too small to cause any detectable desaturation). However, if the left SVC is persistent, as is often the case, then this flow must be rerouted to the systemic venous circulation. If there is a good-sized innominate vein connecting the two SVCs, the left SVC can be ligated immediately below the innominate vein. However, in the absence of an innominate vein, the left SVC should be baffled into the RA either by rerooting the CS with a long oval-shaped patch placed into the left atrium to baffle left SVC flow through the defect in the atrial septum. Alternatively, if there is a good-sized right atrial appendage, the left SVC can be transected and anastomosed into an opening created in the apex at the right appendage. A further alternative is to transect the left SVC and create a left-sided cavo-pulmonary (Glenn) anastomosis.

Complications

In children and young adults, this is low-risk surgery with a peri-operative mortality of less than 0.5 per cent. Residual leaks are rare and can be closed with a device if necessary.

Late serous pericardial effusions are common (up to 15 per cent) and probably reactive in aetiology, related to the sudden decrease in right heart size. Creation of a large pericardial window intra-operatively may reduce this risk.

ASD closure after age 11 predisposes to the development of atrial arrhythmias. Atrial flutter and re-entrant tachycardias may occur around the patch or atriotomy scar. Atrial fibrillation is the dominant arrhythmia in later life, and in untreated ASDs, sick sinus syndromes may develop in later years.

Sinus node dysfunction is reported in up to 55 per cent of patients after superior sinus venosus repair regardless of strategy used, although it is possible that Warden repair is safest.

Outcomes

Survival after interventional or surgical closure of all ASDs is now greater than 99 per cent. In older age groups, the risks are slightly higher, depending on the degree of right heart failure. However, if pulmonary vascular resistance is normal or even slightly raised at the time of surgery, the results in even older age groups show both symptomatic relief and improved life expectancy.

Further Reading

Amin Z, Hijazi ZM, Bass JL et al. Erosion of Amplazer septal occlude device after closure of secundum atrial septal defects: review of registry of complications and recommendations to minimize future risk. *Cathet Cardiovasc Intervent* 2004; **63**: 496–502.

Campbell M. Natural history of atrial septal defect. *Br Heart J* 1870; **32**: 820–26.

Carroll JD, Carroll EP. Is patent foramen ovale closure indicated for migraine? PFO closure is not indicated for migraine: 'Don't shoot first, ask questions later'. *Circ Cardiovasc Intervent* 2009; **2**: 475–81.

Craig RJ, Selzer A. Natural history and prognosis of atrial septal defect. *Circulation* 1968; **37**: 805–15.

Konstandinides S, Geibel A, Olschewski M et al. A comparison of surgical and medical therapy for atrial septal defect in adults. *N Engl J Med* 1995; **333**: 469–73.

Murphy JG, Gersh BJ, McGoon MD et al. Long-term outcome after surgical repair of isolated atrial septal defect: follow-up at 27 to 32 years. *N Engl J Med* 1990; **323**: 1645–50.

Chapter

8

Anomalous Pulmonary Venous Connection and Cor Triatriatum

Natasha Khan

Introduction

Anomalous pulmonary venous connection is categorized according to whether or not the entire pulmonary venous return is anomalous (total) or only partly anomalous, with some of the venous drainage being normal (partial).

Total Anomalous Pulmonary Venous Connection (TAPVC)

This is also called 'total anomalous pulmonary venous drainage' (TAPVD). The entire pulmonary venous return drains to the right side of the heart or the systemic venous system, usually via a common pulmonary venous confluence. An atrial communication is therefore essential to allow left ventricular filling. It makes up 1 to 2 per cent of congenital heart defects and occurs as in combination with other anomalies in one-third of cases.

Morphology

In most cases the pulmonary veins drain into an extra-cardiac chamber called the 'pulmonary venous confluence', which is a remnant of the embryo's common

pulmonary vein. This confluence drains through a separate channel into the systemic venous circulation.

There are four types of TAPVC:

Supra-cardiac. This is the commonest variant (45 to 55 per cent of TAPVCs), a connection of the pulmonary venous confluence via a vertical vein into the superior vena cava (SVC), the innominate vein or, rarely, the azygous vein. The confluence is horizontally oriented, lying immediately behind the pericardium, facing the back of the left atrium.

Cardiac. Here drainage is directly into the coronary sinus (10 to 15 per cent of TAPVCs).

Infra-diaphragmatic. The pulmonary venous confluence lies posterior to the pericardium behind the heart and drains via a descending vertical vein, through the diaphragm, into the portal circulation or the inferior vena cava (IVC; 20 to 25 per cent of TAPVCs). The orientation of the confluence is vertical rather than horizontal.

Mixed. This involves combinations of the above (5 to 10 per cent), typically with a confluence of the majority of the veins with one or two separate vein(s) draining directly into the SVC or innominate vein.

The common forms are shown in Figure 8.1.

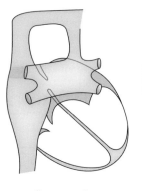 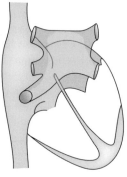 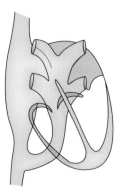

Supra-cardiac   Cardiac   Infra-cardiac

Figure 8.1 Diagrams showing the common patterns of total anomalous pulmonary venous drainage.

Pathophysiology

The venous return from the pulmonary circulation drains to the right side of the heart (causing obligate mixing of the venous circulations and cyanosis), resulting in right heart volume loading, and the pre-load to the left side of the heart is entirely dependent on the atrial communication. Any restriction of the atrial communication causes further right heart pressure loading with under-filling of the left heart and poor systemic perfusion.

Furthermore, if there is any obstruction to the pulmonary venous return into the systemic circulation, then there will be venous congestion in the lungs and pulmonary oedema, setting up a potentially lethal combination of profound cyanosis, pulmonary hypertension and poor systemic cardiac output. More severe degrees of obstruction are associated with lymphatic abnormalities within the lungs.

Obstruction is most commonly seen in infra-cardiac types (most have some degree of obstruction), where the draining vein is obstructed in its passage through the liver. Less severe degrees of obstruction can be seen with (~50 per cent of) supra-cardiac types, where the draining vein can get trapped in the 'vice' between bronchus and pulmonary artery. Obstruction does not occur with cardiac types.

Any obstruction is usually at the level of the draining vein, but sometimes the individual veins themselves can be narrowed, particularly in the infra-cardiac group. Isolated pulmonary vein stenosis carries a particularly poor prognosis.

Presentation

If there is obstruction to pulmonary venous return, presentation is at birth with respiratory distress, cyanosis and collapse. Symptoms develop within 24 hours of birth, and death occurs without treatment in the first weeks of life.

In the absence of pulmonary venous obstruction, patients present in early infancy with variable degrees of cyanosis and right heart volume overload. There may be dyspnoea, failure to thrive, and recurrent chest infections. The degree of cyanosis can be relatively mild if there is unobstructed return.

Severity of symptoms depends on the degree of obstruction, but severe cases can present in extremis with profound cyanosis and require resuscitation and emergency surgery. ECG shows right ventricular hypertrophy.

CXR in obstructed cases shows plethoric and congested lung fields with a relatively small heart shadow; the venous obstruction creates a characteristic 'ground glass' pattern to the lung fields. In unobstructed cases, there tends to be cardiomegaly with less pulmonary plethora.

Echocardiography is diagnostic and demonstrates the absence of pulmonary venous connections to the left atrium in combination with right-to-left shunting across the atrial septal defect (ASD). The positions of all four veins should be identified. There is right ventricular and pulmonary artery volume loading. The left ventricle often appears small, but this is due to under-filling and compression from the enlarged right side – it is seldom due to inadequate development – and the aortic and mitral dimensions are normal.

CT scan and MRI are rarely necessary but can be used to further delineate the anatomy if there are doubts on echocardiography on the position of individual veins. Cardiac catheterization is not necessary.

Management

Management depends on the presentation. In obstructed TAPVC, the patient usually presents shocked, cyanotic and acidotic. This type of patient must be stabilized as much as possible with intubation, ventilation with 100 per cent oxygen and/or nitric oxide, prostaglandin infusion, inotropic support and correction of acidosis. The definitive treatment is surgical, and this must be undertaken emergently.

In unobstructed TAPVC there is no immediate urgency, and elective surgery can be planned before six months of age. Patients with minor degrees of obstruction usually have a degree of right heart failure and should be repaired as a priority.

Surgery

This is the only treatment for TAPVC, and the aim is to redirect pulmonary venous flow to the left atrium. Surgery is performed using moderate hypothermia and bicaval cannulation or with deep hypothermic arrest, according to preference – although the latter may be necessary in newborn obstructive cases where collateral return otherwise prevents an adequate view.

In infra- and supra-cardiac TAPVC, redirection can be achieved by laying open the confluence where it sits behind the pericardium, making a matching incision into the posterior wall of the left atrium/appendage and anastomosing the two together. The draining vein can be ligated (some recommend

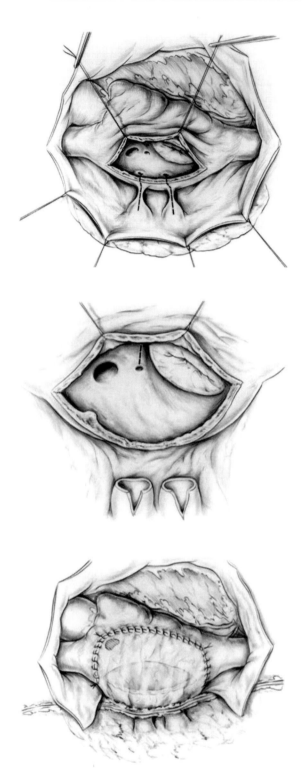

Figure 8.2 'Sutureless' repair technique for recurrent pulmonary vein stenosis.
Source: From Lacour-Gayet F. Surgery for pulmonary venous obstruction after repair of total anomalous pulmonary venous return. *Semin Thorac Cardiovasc Surg Pediatr Card Surg Annu* 2006; 45–50.

leaving this open in case recurrent obstruction occurs) and the ASD/PFO closed. Various approaches can be used, either dislocating the heart out of the pericardium or leaving the heart in position and cutting through the right atrium, across the septum and through the posterior wall of the left atrium. Alternatively, the confluence can be approached working between the aorta and SVC to access the posterior pericardium.

In cardiac TAPVC, the atrial septum can be partially resected, the coronary sinus unroofed back into the left atrium to create a large opening and a patch used to close the atrial septum, committing all the coronary sinus return into the left atrium (LA). This will inevitably also direct the coronary venous return to the LA, but this right-to-left shunt is small and not clinically significant.

Postoperative Management. Obstructed cases will have varying degrees of pulmonary hypertension pre-operatively and are at risk of pulmonary hypertensive crises postoperatively: a direct pulmonary artery (PA) pressure monitoring line can be helpful to direct inhaled nitric oxide (iNO) treatment if required. Since the left ventricle has been relatively under-filled , the sudden increase in preload can reveal a non-compliant left ventricle (LV) that is sensitive to volume changes, and monitoring LA pressure is also useful.

Recurrent Obstruction. This can occur in 10 to 15 per cent, most commonly in the infra-cardiac group, and it tends to occur within the first six months. It can occur either at the anastomotic site or within the veins themselves. Significant obstruction needs surgical revision. Stenoses involving the origin of the pulmonary veins are best managed using a 'sutureless' technique that opens the vein into the pericardium and closes the atrium to the surrounding pericardium, avoiding having to place any sutures in the vein itself (Figure 8.2). The success of this technique has now been extended in some centres to primary repair of TAPVC to try to avoid trauma to the pulmonary vein intima.

Outcomes. Obstructed neonates can be at very high risk, carrying a mortality as high as 15 to 20 per cent. The risk in the remainder of cases is 2 to 5 per cent depending on age, weight, single-ventricle anatomy and degree of obstruction.

The mortality of surgical re-intervention for recurrent obstruction is 15 to 25 per cent, with risk factors being early representation and stenosis within the individual veins rather than at the atrial level.

Cor Triatriatum

This is a rare anomaly (0.1 per cent of congenital cardiac malformations) in which there is a diaphragm sitting within the LA, dividing it into two chambers: the pulmonary veins drain into an antechamber separated from the true LA by this diaphragm, giving the heart the appearance of having three atria. If there is any degree of obstruction at the level of the diaphragm, then the presentation is similar to that of obstructed TAPVC. The condition can occur in isolation or in association with VSD, tetralogy of Fallot or partial anomalous pulmonary venous drainage. The anomaly is generally seen within the LA (hence the term 'cor triatriatum sinister') but has very rarely been described within the right atrium ('cor triatriatum dextre')

Morphology

The pulmonary veins drain into the posterior left atrial 'antechamber', separated from the true left atrium by a fibromuscular diaphragm. The right atrium may communicate with one or both chambers. The true LA contains the left atrial appendage and the mitral valve. In 75 per cent of cases, the connection between the pulmonary venous collecting chamber and the LA is restrictive. If the opening is unrestrictive, then the lesion has no haemodynamic consequences.

Presentation

When there is obstruction to pulmonary venous flow, the presentation is early with pulmonary venous congestion and pulmonary arterial hypertension, with an urgency for surgical repair. If there is good communication from the antechamber to the RA, then there will be less congestion of the lungs but more volume loading of the right heart, with venous mixing leading to some cyanosis. These patients may present as adults.

Echocardiography is diagnostic, and care should be taken to delineate all four pulmonary veins. The position of any interatrial communications and direction of flow must be carefully documented. Echo should differentiate this from supra-mitral membrane, where the membrane lies between the mitral valve and the left atrial appendage (LAA), whereas in cor triatriatum the mitral valve and the LAA are on the same side of the membrane.

Management

If the patient presents acutely with pulmonary venous obstruction, the aim of management is to stabilize the patient with a view to performing surgery urgently. When there is good communication across the diaphragm, elective repair is sufficient.

Surgery

Surgical repair is required for all obstructed cases. The RA is opened, and the PFO/ASD is enlarged to allow access to the LA. The diaphragm is then resected and the atrial septum closed with a patch. Care has to be taken when entering the chamber as the anatomy can be deceiving, and it is essential to identify the position of the pulmonary veins and the mitral valve before resecting the membrane.

Outcomes

The outcome from surgery depends on the degree of obstruction and any associated defects, and therefore, in published series, mortality ranges from 3 to 20 per cent. Long-term outcome after repair is excellent, and recurrent obstruction is very rare, since the pulmonary veins themselves are not involved in the surgery.

Partially Anomalous Pulmonary Venous Drainage (PAPVD)

This is a rare congenital cardiac defect in which some of the pulmonary veins (most commonly from the right lung) are connected to the right atrium or systemic veins rather than to the left atrium. Occasionally, all the veins from one lung may drain anomalously, but more commonly, a single pulmonary vein is anomalous. The most common form is in combination with a sinus venosus ASD in which a number of right-sided pulmonary veins connect to the SVC or RA (80 per cent of all PAPVDs; see above). Anomalous left-sided veins can drain into the innominate vein, coronary sinus, left subclavian vein or even the RA atrium or SVC.

Scimitar Syndrome. This consists of PAPVD of the right pulmonary veins draining into the IVC (the 'scimitar' sign created by this large venous channel curving around the RA to reach the IVC). This is associated with pulmonary arterial anomalies to the supply to the right lung – typically the right lower lobe supplied by a collateral vessel from the abdominal

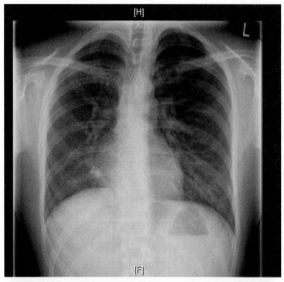

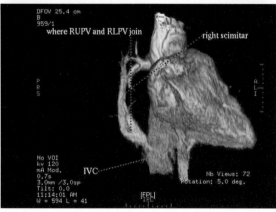

Figure 8.3 CXR and MRI reconstruction in scimitar syndrome showing the right pulmonary veins draining thought the 'scimitar' channel to the IVC. (A black-and-white version of this figure will appear in some formats. For the colour version, please refer to the plate section.)

aorta, but arterial supply can be normal. There are also associated bronchial anomalies with sequestered lobe(s), but again, the lung can be normal (Figure 8.3).

Pathophysiology and Natural History

PAPVD causes a left-to-right shunt, the magnitude of which depends on the number of veins that drain anomalously. A single anomalous vein is rarely haemodynamically significant. The pathophysiology is similar to an ASD in isolated PAPVD and otherwise depending on associated anomalies. The long-term complications of arrhythmias, right-sided heart failure and pulmonary vascular disease are only seen in adults.

Presentation and Examination

Isolated PAPVD is often asymptomatic, but larger shunts present in a similar way to ASD. Adults may become symptomatic from chronic right-sided volume overload, with palpitations, dyspnoea and chest pain. The presentation of scimitar syndrome depends on the degree of pulmonary hypoplasia.

Imaging

Echocardiography. Even with careful echocardiography, isolated PAPVC can be missed if there is not a high index of suspicion. In adults, contrast echocardiography may help with the diagnosis, and trans-oesophageal echo (TOE) may delineate the pulmonary venous anatomy better. Right ventricular dilatation may be the only abnormality seen initially.

MRI/CT. These are useful where PAPVC is suspected to further define the exact pulmonary venous anatomy.

Cardiac catheter. This is rarely necessary but may be used in an adult to evaluate right-sided pressures and exclude associated coronary artery disease. The pulmonary-to-systemic blood flow ratio Qp:Qs can be exactly calculated to help in surgical decision-making.

Surgery

If the Qp:Qs is greater than 1.5:1, surgical therapy in children is justified. In adults, assessment of pulmonary vasculature must be undertaken to guide the decision to undertake surgical correction.

Repair is usually performed through a median sternotomy, using cardiopulmonary bypass, but as with ASDs, less invasive incisions/approaches have been attempted. The majority of PAPVDs repaired are those associated with a sinus venosus ASD, as described earlier.

There are two methods for surgical repair:

Tunnelling/Intra-atrial Baffling. The RA is opened, and the ASD is closed with a patch baffling the right pulmonary veins into the left atrium. If the ASD is small or absent, the atrial septum is opened in such a way as to create a flap of septal tissue, which can then be sutured to the lateral wall to baffle the pulmonary veins posteriorly into the LA. This flap can be augmented, or replaced, with a patch of autologous pericardium.

Re-implantation. The anomalous veins can be ligated and divided and then reanastomosed to the LA. The vein may be anastomosed to the LA in a side-to-side fashion for a long anastomosis or in an end-to-side fashion with a wide, spatulated anastomosis. Anomalous left veins draining into the innominate vein can be re-implanted into the left atrial appendage. This procedure can be performed through a left thoracotomy without cardiopulmonary bypass.

Outcomes

Outcomes for repair in children are excellent, with good long-term freedom from arrhythmias. There is a risk of late pulmonary vein stenosis in any baffled channel or at re-implantation suture lines, usually amenable to interventional balloon. In adults presenting with arrhythmias, concomitant maze should be performed, but persistent atrial fibrillation (AF) is common, and there may be continuing right ventricular dysfunction after surgery.

Current surgical mortality after repair of scimitar syndrome is less than 5 per cent, with a 10 per cent incidence of pulmonary vein stenosis, more likely with baffling techniques as compared to re-implantation.

Further Reading

Fragata J, Magalhães M, Baquero L et al. Partial anomalous pulmonary venous connections: surgical management. *Pediatr Congenital Heart Surg* 2013; **4**(1): 44–49.

Hörer J, Neuray C, Vogt M et al. What to expect after repair of total anomalous pulmonary venous connection: data from 193 patients and 2902 patient years. *Eur J Cardiothorac Surg* 2013; **44**(5): 800–7.

Lo Rito M, Gazzaz T, Wilder T et al. Repair type influences mode of pulmonary vein stenosis in total anomalous pulmonary venous drainage. *Ann Thorac Surg* 2015; **100**(2): 654–62.

Saxena P, Burkhart HM, Schaff HV et al. Surgical repair of cor triatriatum sinister: the Mayo Clinic 50-year experience. *Ann Thorac Surg* 2014; **97**(5): 1659–56.

Ungerleider RM, Pasquali SK, Welke KF et al. Contemporary patterns of surgery and outcomes for aortic coarctation: an analysis of the Society of Thoracic Surgeons Congenital Heart Surgery Database. *J Thorac Cardiovasc Surg* 2013; **145**(1): 150–57.

Vida VL, Padalino MA, Boccuzzo G et al. Scimitar syndrome: a European Congenital Heart Surgeons Association (ECHSA) multicentric study. *Circulation* 2010; **122**(12): 1159–66.

Yun TJ, Coles JG, Konstantinov IE et al. Conventional and sutureless techniques for management of the pulmonary veins: evolution of indications from postrepair pulmonary vein stenosis to primary pulmonary vein anomalies. *J Thorac Cardiovasc Surg* 2005; **129**(1): 167–74.

Ventricular Septal Defects

Natasha Khan

Introduction

Ventricular septal defects (VSDs) are the commonest congenital heart defect, accounting for 25 to 30 per cent of all congenital heart disease. However, the majority are small defects that either close spontaneously or are of no clinical significance. The clinical implications depend on their size, number and location in the ventricular septum. They occur as isolated lesions or in combination with other anomalies. They are the commonest cardiac defect found in chromosomal abnormalities such as trisomies 13, 18 and 21 and 22q11 deletion, but 95 per cent of VSDs are found in patients with normal chromosomes.

Morphology

From a surgical standpoint, the location of a VSD is important as it defines the approach to closing it and alerts the surgeon as to the location of conduction fibres that may be damaged when closing the VSD.

VSDs can most simply be classified as follows (Figures 9.1 to 9.3):

Peri-membranous VSDs. These occur where a margin of the VSD consists of fibrous continuity between the tricuspid and aortic valves. The conduction bundles run along the inferior rim of the defect. They may be inlet, outlet or inlet-outlet VSDs. They account for about 80 per cent of VSDs, requiring surgical closure in some series. They may cause aortic valve regurgitation secondary to right or non–coronary cusp prolapse into the defect. (They are also called 'infracristal' or 'membranous'.)

Juxta-arterial or Doubly Committed Sub-arterial VSDs. These occur where the conjoined leaflets of the aortic and pulmonary valves form the rim of the VSD. The conduction bundles are remote from the defect. (They are also called 'supracristal', 'conal' or 'infundibular'.) They may also cause aortic insufficiency by right coronary cusp prolapse. They

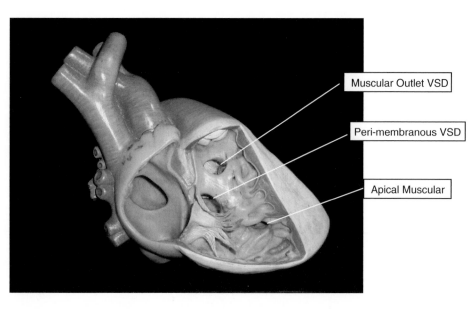

Muscular Outlet VSD

Peri-membranous VSD

Apical Muscular

Figure 9.1 3D model of the heart with the free wall of the right atrium and ventricle removed. Arrows show the positions of commonly occurring VSDs. (A black-and-white version of this figure will appear in some formats. For the colour version, please refer to the plate section.)

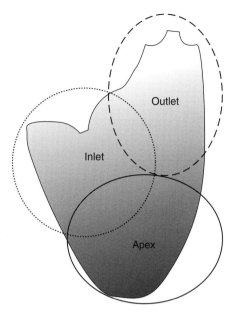

Figure 9.2 Representation of the ventricular septum viewed from the right ventricular side. The areas of the septum can be approximately divided into three regions: the inlet portion, below the level of the tricuspid valve; the outlet portion, above the level of the tricuspid valve; and the apical trabecular area.

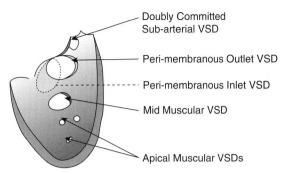

Figure 9.3 The ventricular septum viewed from the right ventricular side showing the positions of commonly found VSDs.

constitute about 5 per cent of VSDs seen in the West but are more common in Asian countries. They do not close spontaneously.

Muscular VSDs. These are the commonest type of VSD, and most close spontaneously. The rims of the VSD are entirely muscular, and they can occur anywhere within the ventricular septum, being described by their position as inlet, apicotrabecular or outlet defects. They can be multiple. The conduction bundles are remote from the defect, and in the case of the inlet VSD, they run near the superior margin of the defect. Larger defects may require surgical closure, accounting for 5 to 10 per cent of VSDs closed surgically.

Pathophysiology and Natural History

Restrictive defect. Small defects presenting resistance to flow across the defect, with pulmonary-to-systemic blood flow ratio Qp:Qs < 1.5.

Non-restrictive Defect. This occurs where the cross-sectional area of the defect is equivalent to or larger than that of the aortic annulus. There is no resistance to flow across the defect, the right and left ventricular pressures approach parity and the Qp:Qs is inversely proportional to the ratio of the pulmonary-to-systemic vascular resistances.

Haemodynamic Consequences of a Non-restrictive Defect. The magnitude and direction of shunting across the defect depend on the size of the defect and the compliance of the distal vascular bed. The left-to-right shunt causes increased pulmonary blood flow ('pulmonary over-circulation') and left ventricular volume overload leading to congestive cardiac failure.

Neonates and infants with unrestrictive defects present in heart failure and require urgent repair; if untreated, the one-year survival is only 10 per cent. At the other end of the spectrum, small, restrictive defects are of no haemodynamic significance and cause no symptoms. Larger defects that escape detection can lead to irreversible pulmonary hypertension and pulmonary vascular disease in the long term. In untreated patients, the raised pulmonary vascular resistance and high right-sided pressures can lead to shunt reversal and cyanosis in about 10 per cent of these patients in the third and fourth decades (Eisenmenger syndrome).

Over 80 per cent of muscular defects close spontaneously by the age of four years, as do 30 to 40 per cent of (smaller) peri-membranous defects. Inlet VSDs and doubly committed sub-arterial VSDs do not tend to close spontaneously. Small, restrictive VSDs should not affect prognosis but do carry a slightly increased risk of bacterial endocarditis, and even small peri-membranous VSDs may cause aortic cusp prolapse and evolving aortic regurgitation.

Presentation

Larger defects present in infancy with congestive cardiac failure, recurrent chest infections, failure to thrive and breathlessness. A Qp:Qs > 2 is poorly tolerated. Symptoms usually begin as pulmonary vascular resistance falls in the four to six weeks after birth – babies may be sweaty and tachypnoeic during feeds, unable to finish adequate volumes of feed, and fail to gain adequate weight. Smaller defects may be entirely asymptomatic. Infective endocarditis is a risk of VSD. Doubly committed sub-arterial (DCSA) and outlet peri-membranous VSDs may present with aortic regurgitation, with the right coronary cusp (RCC0 prolapsing through the VSD. Many asymptomatic children present with murmurs. It is rare for adults to present with unknown significant VSD.

The ECG can be normal, but larger defects may show left and right ventricular hypertrophy. Inferior-axis deviation is seen in some inlet VSDs. CXR shows cardiomegaly and increased vascular markings. Echocardiography is the definitive investigation and is diagnostic, defines the location and size of the defect, the extent of the haemodynamic consequences and associated anomalies.

Cardiac catheterization is not required for the routine investigation of VSDs in infants. In children over one year of age with moderate or unrestrictive VSDs, cardiac catheterization may be required to investigate the pulmonary vascular resistance and the appropriateness of VSD closure. Pulmonary vascular resistance (PVR) of 2 to 4 Wood units indexed can be considered normal. If PVR is 4 to 8 Wood units indexed, but reversible with pulmonary vasodilatation, surgery can be performed. If PVR is greater than 8 Wood units and irreversible with supplemental oxygen and nitric oxide, pulmonary vascular disease is established and irreversible – closing the VSD does not alter the natural history and may lead to higher right ventricular pressures and right ventricular failure.

Indications for surgery are listed in Table 9.1, the majority being neonates or infants with unrestrictive defects who are in some degree of congestive cardiac failure. Primary surgical repair for isolated VSD is the treatment of choice, although pulmonary artery banding is occasionally used in specific circumstances, as an interim 'palliative' procedure (see Table 9.2).

Closure of VSDs

Interventional. Some VSDs can be closed by percutaneously placed devices – these are mainly used to close muscular defects, particularly apical defects that are inaccessible to the surgeon. However, this is mostly restricted to older children as adequate

Table 9.1 Indications for Closing a VSD

- Any unrestrictive defect in a neonate or infant
- Large defect with evidence of congestive heart failure unresponsive to medical therapy
- Qp:Qs > 1.5:1
- Sub-arterial defect causing aortic valve prolapse and regurgitation
- Proven episode of infective endocarditis

Table 9.2 Indications for Pulmonary Artery Banding in the Setting of VSD

- Multiple muscular VSDs
- Larger defects in small neonates with significant co-morbidities (e.g. intercurrent infection)
- Straddle of A-V valves or evidence of ventricular imbalance with concern over size of LV
- In association with coarctation, where coarctation repair is performed through left thoracotomy

vascular access is not possible in smaller infants. Some smaller peri-membranous defects may also be closed in this way, but the proximity of the aortic valve and absence of a 'rim' superiorly to seat the device limit the application – there is also a risk of A-V node block and aortic regurgitation (~5 per cent) and tricuspid regurgitation (~10 per cent).

Surgical. The standard approach in infants and small children is via a median sternotomy using bicaval cannulation, moderate hypothermia and cardioplegic arrest. The majority are approached via the right atrium, working through the tricuspid valve ('trans-atrial repair').

Peri-membranous Defects. These are approached through a right atriotomy. The septal leaflet of the tricuspid valve may have to be retracted gently or even detached for exposure of the VSD. Gore-Tex, Dacron or glutaraldehyde-preserved bovine pericardium is used to close the defect; even small defects should be closed with a patch. Care must be taken to avoid the conduction tissue running along the postero-inferior margin of the VSD (to the surgeon's right hand) by moving the sutures away from the margin. Patches can be placed with continuous or interrupted sutures.

Muscular Defects. Inlet and trabecular muscular defects are approached as earlier through the right atrium. Apical trabecular muscular defects may need to be approached through a right ventriculotomy. Moderate to large defects should be closed with a patch, but smaller defects can be closed with buttressed sutures. Take care to avoid the conduction bundles running along the superior margins of inlet VSDs (left hand of surgeon).

Doubly Committed Sub-arterial (DCSA) Defects. These are most easily approached through a pulmonary arteriotomy, across the pulmonary valve, with some sutures anchoring the patch through the base of pulmonary valve leaflets. The conduction axis is remote from the margins.

If there is associated mild aortic regurgitation, the aortic valve can be left alone, but if the regurgitation is moderate, aortic valve repair should be attempted, plicating or re-suspending the prolapsing leaflet.

Hybrid approaches can be used for suitable mid-muscular defects, delivering a device via a purse-string on the right ventricular surface through which a guide wire, sheath and loading sheath are positioned under trans-oesophageal echo (TOE) guidance.

Complications

Mortality is now less than 1 per cent in isolated VSD but can be higher in multiple defects or when associated with other lesions. Residual VSDs can occur due to either incomplete closure or stitches tearing through the septum under tension. These may need reintervention if the Qp:Qs > 1.5:1.

Conduction Disturbance. Right bundle branch block (RBBB) is almost always seen after peri-membranous VSD closure, but complete heart block occurs in only 1 per cent. In the long term, up to 4 per cent of repaired VSDs can develop sick sinus syndrome.

Prophylactic antibiotics (to cover an invasive procedure or dental work) are recommended for only the first six months after surgery. Aortic and tricuspid valve regurgitation can occur if these structures are damaged during closure, reinforcing the importance of performing intra-operative echo to exclude these problems.

Follow-up

All children should be followed up to ensure return of normal ventricular dimensions and exclude residual lesions or development of aortic regurgitation. Children who have no residual issues can be discharged.

Further Reading

Corone P, Doyon F, Gaudeau S et al. Natural history of ventricular septal defect: a study involving 790 cases. *Circulation* 1977; **55**(6): 908–15.

Predescu D, Chaturvedi RR, Friedberg MK et al. Complete heart block associated with device closure of perimembranous ventricular septal defects. *J Thorac Cardiovasc Surg* 2008; **136**(5): 1223–28.

Yip WC, Zimmerman F, Hijazi ZM. Heart block and empirical therapy after transcatheter closure of perimembranous ventricular septal defect. *Cathet Cardiovasc Intervent* 2005; **66**(3): 436–41.

Atrio-ventricular Septal Defects

Chapter 10

David J. Barron

Introduction

This group of defects is characterized by a defect in the centre of the heart (the atrio-ventricular junction) with a single valve structure straddling the centre of the heart. Thus there is no true mitral or tricuspid valve; rather there is a left and right component of the common valve which is made up a mural leaflets and bridging leaflets – so called as they bridge the ventricular septum (Figure 10.1). Overall they account for 4 to 5 per cent of all congenital heart disease. The defects are strongly associated with Down syndrome, accounting for up to 80 per cent of all complete atrio-ventricular septal defects (AVSDs) in the United Kingdom (40 per cent of all Down syndrome

cases have an AVSD). These defects have also been called 'endocardial cushion defects', reflecting their embryological development, and 'A-V canal defects', which, although still used, is not morphologically correct.

Morphology. There is a spectrum of disease that most importantly focuses on the extent of the VSD component: if the VSD is shallow or small, then the bridging leaflets of the valve become fused to the crest of the ventricular septum, obliterating the VSD – thus, the only defect is above the valve at the atrial level in the form of a primum ASD. This is referred to as a 'partial AVSD' (although also called 'primum ASD'). However, with larger VSD components, there is a defect both below and above the A-V valve creating a 'complete AVSD', with the VSD having a characteristic semi-circular shape and involving the peri-membranous septum, extending from the inlet to the outlet. Occasionally, the result is an 'intermediate AVSD', where the majority of the VSD component has been sealed off by the A-V valve tissue but there is still a small shunt at the ventricular level where the bridging leaflets gape at their meeting point in the middle of the defect. The valve morphology is extremely variable, particularly in the septal attachments of the superior bridging leaflet (defined by the Rastelli classification), and the leaflets themselves are variable in both number and quality, which can lead to varying degrees of valvar incompetence. Rarely there can be associated right ventricular outflow tract (RVOT) obstruction with deviation of the outlet septum creating 'AVSD/Fallot'.

Pathophysiology and Presentation. These depend on the extent of the VSD component and the degree of associated A-V valve incompetence. Large defects create a significant ventricular shunt with volume loading of the circulation and congestive cardiac failure with pulmonary plethora. The volume load on the heart is exacerbated by

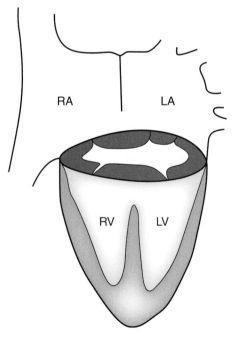

Figure 10.1 Anatomy of a complete atrio-ventricular septal defect. There is a single valve structure straddling the heart made up of mural leaflets and bridging leaflets. There is a ventricular septal defect below the valve and a primum atrial septal defect above it.

any associated A-V valve regurgitation. These lesions have a tendency to develop early pulmonary vascular hypertension if untreated, particularly in association with Down syndrome. Thus, presentation is usually in early infancy or the neonatal period with heart failure, tachypnoea and failure to thrive. In contrast, the haemodynamic lesion in partial AVSD is an atrial shunt, and as with other ASDs, these rarely produce symptoms in childhood. However, if there is associated A-V valve regurgitation, this can cause congestive heart failure. AVSD/Fallot may be a more balanced lesion, the RVOT obstruction protecting from heart failure – but it may produce cyanosis and spelling depending on the degree of obstruction (see Chapter 11).

Investigation. Clinical examination will reveal signs of congestive heart failure depending on the severity of the defect. Murmurs of A-V valve regurgitation may be present. The ECG shows a characteristic superior-axis pattern (extreme left-axis deviation, which reflects the deviation of the conduction system by the defect), and CXR shows cardiomegaly and pulmonary plethora in a complete defect. Echocardiography is the most useful investigation, and further imaging is not usually required. It is important to assess the morphology and function of the A-V valves carefully to inform the surgical repair.

Initial Management and Surgery

Heart failure should be treated with diuretics and angiotensin-converting enzyme (ACE) inhibitors, particularly if there is significant A-V valve regurgitation. Large defects can be difficult to manage medically, and any intercurrent chest infection can result in rapid deterioration. Complete defects should undergo surgical repair within the first three months of life. Delaying longer, even when the baby is managing well, increases the risk of pulmonary vascular disease. Partial AVSDs are usually well tolerated, and surgical repair can be planned electively, usually before school age at three to four years. However, those with significant A-V valve regurgitation may require repair sooner.

Complete surgical repair is the treatment of choice, but initial pulmonary artery banding can be considered if there are important co-morbidities such as intercurrent chest infections or in low-birth-weight babies. The additional afterload of the PA band may potentially worsen A-V valve regurgitation, but

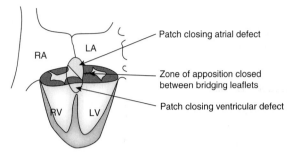

Figure 10.2 Repair of complete AVSD using two-patch technique (RA = right atrium; LA = left atrium; RV = right ventricle; LV = left ventricle).

usually the primary cause of heart failure in AVSD is the large VSD component, and the PA band will reduce this volume load and so actually reduce the regurgitation.

Surgical Repair. Several techniques have been described, but the standard repair for complete AVSD requires a two-patch technique, performed trans-atrially and using a semi-circular patch to close the VSD and a second semi-circular patch to close the primum ASD, sandwiching the bridging leaflets of the A-V valve between them (Figure 10.2). This septates the valve into left and right components, but each must be carefully assessed to achieve competence, usually closing the zone of apposition of the bridging leaflets on the left side to create a single 'septal' leaflet. Accurate repair in choosing the correct position to partition the valve is essential to creating a good long-term result. Finally, the atrial patch completes closure of the primum defect. Many surgeons leave the coronary sinus behind the patch draining into the left atrium in order to ensure that the suture line is well away from the A-V node. This creates a small right-to-left shunt but is not of clinical significance. However, if there are bilateral superior venae cavae (SVCs), then the coronary sinus must be committed to the right atrium as it carries the left SVC flow (the large size of the coronary sinus in this setting allows for the suture line to run into the floor of the sinus and so avoid the conduction in this way). A left atrial pressure monitoring line is valuable in postoperative management.

If the VSD component is relatively shallow, or if there are multiple chordal attachments to the crest of the septum, then it may be possible to close the AVSD with a single patch above the valve. Interrupted sutures are placed through the ventricular septum, through the partition points of the bridging leaflets and then into the patch, sealing the bridging leaflets down onto the crest of the septum from above. The single-patch technique was described by Nunn et al. in Brisbane with excellent outcomes, but care has to be taken when there is a large outlet component to the VSD that the technique does not close down the left outflow tract behind the superior bridging leaflet.

Partial AVSDs are repaired with a single atrial patch. Since the A-V valve tissue itself forms part of the margin of the defect, sutures are usually passed from beneath the valve tissue (on the ventricular side) to secure the patch to the A-V valve. Again, the valve must be carefully assessed, and the zone of apposition between the bridging leaflets (which has the appearance of a 'cleft', although morphologically it is not) should be closed. The coronary sinus can be left behind the patch, just as described earlier.

Hospital mortality for complete AVSD repair is 3 to 4 per cent. This is significantly higher than for isolated VSD repair, reflecting the complex nature of the surgery and the fact that the patients are usually in significant heart failure preoperatively. Postoperative complications include a risk of heart block of 1 to 2 per cent and the risk of residual left (and right) A-V valve regurgitation. Pulmonary hypertensive crises are now rare as long as repair is performed early (<3 months) but used to be much commoner when repair was performed later. Mortality for partial AVSD is under 1 per cent, reflecting that these are generally older children who have not been in significant heart failure.

The commonest late problems involve the development or progression of A-V valve regurgitation, requiring further repair or replacement; 10 to 20 per cent of all patients are over age 20. This reflects the fact that the A-V valves in AVSD are very different from normal mitral valve with abnormal chordal attachments, irregular and dysplastic leaflets. The common A-V valve junction in AVSD results in the aortic root being 'unwedged' and sitting further away from the A-V junction than in the normal heart. This can lead to a slightly longer and narrower left outflow tract ('gooseneck' LVOT) than in the normal heart and a higher incidence of developing late sub-aortic stenosis.

Further Reading

Backer CL, Stewart RD, Mavroudis C. Overview: history, anatomy, timing, and results of complete atrioventricular canal. *Semin Thorac Cardiovasc Surg Pediatr Card Surg Annu* 2007: 3–10.

Bakhtiary F, Takacs J, Cho MY et al. Long-term results after repair of complete atrioventricular septal defect with two-patch technique *Ann Thorac Surg* 2010; **89**(4): 1239–43.

Hoohenkerk GJ, Bruggemans EF, Koolbergen DR, Rijlaarsdam ME, Hazekamp MG. Long-term results of reoperation for left atrioventricular valve regurgitation after correction of atrioventricular septal defects *Ann Thorac Surg* 2012; **93**(3): 849–55.

Nunn GR. Atrioventricular canal: modified single patch technique. *Semin Thorac Cardiovasc Surg Pediatr Card Surg Annu* 2007: 28–31.

Pontailler M, Kalfa D, Garcia E et al. Reoperations for left atrioventricular valve dysfunction after repair of atrioventricular septal defect. *Eur J Cardiothorac Surg* 2013;

Tetralogy of Fallot

David J. Barron

Introduction

Tetralogy of Fallot (ToF) is the commonest cyanotic heart condition and accounts for 5 per cent of all congenital heart diseases. The four components are a ventricular septal defect (VSD), overriding aorta, right ventricular outflow tract (RVOT) obstruction and right ventricular hypertrophy (RVH). Morphologically, this can be characterized by an antero-cephalad deviation of the outflow septum that results in a large peri-membranous VSD that is overridden by the aorta and multi-level stenosis of the deviated RVOT. The RVH is the natural response to this outflow tract obstruction (Figure 11.1).

The degree of right ventricular outflow tract (RVOT) obstruction is variable but involves the muscular infundibulum, the pulmonary valve and annulus and the main pulmonary artery and the branch origins. Beyond this, the pulmonary arteries and vasculature are usually normal.

ToF is also associated with right-sided aortic arch (15 per cent), bilateral superior venae cavae (SVCs; 10 per cent) and, as part of the family of cono-truncal anomalies, has an association with DiGeorge syndrome (15 per cent). It can also be associated with other non-cardiac conditions such as vertebral defects, anal atresia, cardiac defects, tracheo-oesophageal fistula, renal anomalies, and limb abnormalities (VACTERL) association and coloboma, heart defects, atresia choanae, growth retardation, genital abnormalities, and ear abnormalities (CHARGE) syndrome. There is a subgroup of (usually more severe) cases in which the aorta is more committed to the right ventricle than it is to the left: in this arrangement, the aorta has moved more anteriorly and is no longer in continuity with the mitral valve. This is a variant of double-outlet right ventricle (DORV) and can be more challenging to repair.

Clinical Presentation. Time of presentation and symptoms will depend upon the degree of RVOT

obstruction, which dictates the degree of cyanosis. Most neonates are acyanotic or only mildly cyanosed but become gradually more cyanosed as the RVH progresses and the degree of RVOT obstruction increases. A newborn who is severely cyanosed will often respond to conservative management using prostaglandin to maintain ductal patency and allow the high pulmonary vascular resistance of the newborn to subside. Infants and older children may develop cyanotic 'spells' that are caused by a temporary dynamic increase in the degree of muscular infundibular obstruction – these may respond to

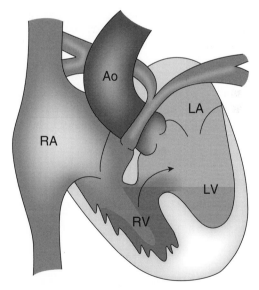

Figure 11.1 (A) The anatomy of tetralogy of Fallot. There is a large ventricular septal defect and multi-level obstruction to the right ventricular outflow tract; this is of a variable degree of severity that consists of muscular obstruction below the valve, valvar stenosis and a small main pulmonary artery. The arrow shows the right-to-left flow across the VSD. (B) Surgical repair of tetralogy of Fallot showing the VSD closed with a patch and the RVOT enlarged with a combination of muscle resection and placement of a trans-annular patch (LV = left ventricle; RV = right ventricle; LA = left atrium; RA = right atrium; Ao = aorta; RVOT = right ventricular outflow tract obstruction).

beta-blocker therapy that helps relax the infundibular myocardium. Children may remain symptom-free for

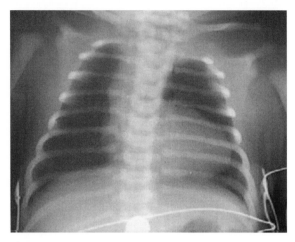

Figure 11.2 CXR in tetralogy of Fallot showing the classic 'boot-shaped heart', which reflects the hypertrophied right ventricle and relatively small main pulmonary artery.

many years if the degree of RVOT obstruction is mild, but the natural history is one of gradual but progressive cyanosis. Heart failure is very rare since the RVOT obstruction protects the lungs from over-circulation despite the large VSD.

Investigation. CXR shows a characteristic boot-shaped heart representing the prominent right ventricle but relatively small main pulmonary arteries (Figure 11.2). ECG will show RVH occasionally with right bundle branch block (RBBB). Echocardiography is the mainstay of investigation (Figure 11.3) and will usually be able to demonstrate all features of the anatomy. Cardiac catheter or CT angiography is sometimes required to delineate the branch pulmonary artery anatomy or to confirm coronary pattern.

Management. The condition is usually relatively stable with a natural history of gradually progressive cyanosis as the RVOT obstruction progresses. Occasionally, severe cases present as newborns or small infants with severe cyanosis requiring

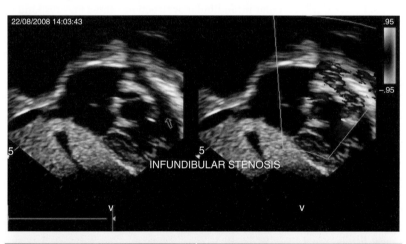

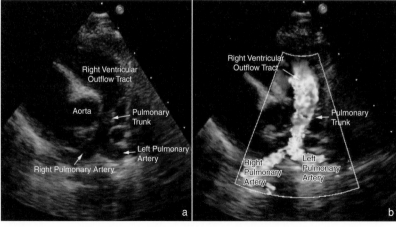

Figure 11.3 Echocardiographic still images of tetralogy of Fallot showing turbulent flow in the long, narrowed right ventricular infundibulum. The lower two images (A and B) show the composite hypoplasia of small infundibulum, valve annulus, and main and branch pulmonary arteries. (A black-and-white version of this figure will appear in some formats. For the colour version, please refer to the plate section.)

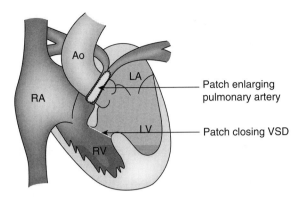

Figure 11.4 Repaired tetralogy of Fallot. The VSD is closed with a prosthetic patch, committing the LV to the aorta. The right outflow tract has been enlarged by resecting muscle bundles and patch enlargement of the pulmonary valve and main pulmonary artery. If the incision crosses the annulus of the valve into the infundibulum, it is referred to as a 'trans-annular patch'.

inpatient treatment, rehydration (if water depleted) and the use of prostaglandin in severe cases. Newborns may settle with this treatment alone as the pulmonary vascular resistance falls over the first days of life and saturations improve. Persistently cyanosed patients require early intervention – this has traditionally been the use of a Blalock-Taussig shunt (see Chapter 4), but primary repair is also feasible in appropriate cases. An alternative is to place a RVOT stent or a small outflow tract patch to improve pulmonary blood flow. The stent is attractive in that it avoids surgery, but it does require considerable skill to deploy in a small baby.

Older infants and children may gradually become more cyanosed but may also develop hypercyanotic 'spells' often triggered by physical exertion or coughing. These are caused by spasm of the infundibular muscle and respond to increasing preload on the heart (i.e. giving volume, although older patients learn strategies to increase their own preload with manoeuvres such as squatting) or the use of beta-blockers to relieve infundibular spasm. Treatment of ToF is usually supportive therapies such as these until the child is referred for elective repair.

Surgical Repair. Anatomical correction is achieved by closing the VSD and relieving any outflow tract obstruction. Performed under moderate hypothermia with bicaval cannulation, the pulmonary arteries should be clearly defined such that any areas of stenosis (usually at their origins) can be addressed. Any

residual patent ductus arteriosus (PDA) is ligated. The VSD can usually be closed trans-atrially with a prosthetic patch, working through the tricuspid valve. Relief of the RVOT obstruction needs careful consideration: obstructive septo-parietal muscle bars in the infundibulum can be divided, and if the cusps of the pulmonary valve are fused, they can be opened with a valvotomy, but if the annulus of the valve is too small, then the incision in the main pulmonary artery needs to be extended across the annulus and a short distance into the infundibulum to allow the outflow tract to open out adequately. The aim should be to ensure that the outflow tract reaches the predicted size for the patients' height/weight (Kirklin tables) or at least within a Z-score of -2. The outflow tract is then repaired with a prosthetic patch – if the annulus is crossed, then this is referred to as a 'trans-annular patch' and will have inevitably rendered the pulmonary valve incompetent (Figure 11.4). Various techniques have been used to re-establish a competent valve in these situations, most commonly by creating a mono-cusp outflow tract patch in two layers or with a mono-cusp patch created from an aortic homograft. These techniques are effective in reducing the amount of pulmonary regurgitation (PR) immediately postoperatively, but most go onto develop significant PR over the following years.

Anatomical Considerations. In hearts with DORV, the access to the VSD margins can be limited from a trans-atrial approach, and it may be necessary to perform a small ventriculotomy to gain adequate access to the superior and lateral margins of the VSD. Similarly, in hearts with a doubly committed component to the VSD, it may be necessary to close the defect from above, working through the trans-annular incision. Presence of an anomalous left anterior descending (LAD) artery requires careful assessment – if the annulus of the valve is adequate, then a trans-atrial, trans-pulmonary repair can be safely performed, but if a trans-annular incision would be required, then it may be better to use an RV-PA conduit to avoid damaging the coronary arteries. In this situation, the native outflow tract remains open, and a separate ventriculotomy is made below the coronary arteries for the conduit, thus creating a 'double-outlet' right ventricle.

Postoperative Management. Problems with right ventricular function are the greatest risk because the procedure involves muscle resection in a hypertrophied ventricle and usually creates some degree of pulmonary incompetence. This can create the substrate for a stiff and 'restrictive' RV with predominantly diastolic dysfunction and consequent low cardiac output, requiring high right atrial pressures. This 'restrictive physiology' is characterized by the transmission of the atrial systolic contraction seen in the pulmonary arteries, reflecting the stiff nature of the RV. It is important to ensure that there is no residual RVOT obstruction as this will exacerbate the problem. The situation usually resolves with supportive therapy, accepting high right atrial pressures and the use of lusitropic inotropes such as milrinone and avoiding drugs that increase myocardial stiffness such as adrenaline where possible. Leaving a small patent foramen ovale (PFO) in Fallot repair has been supported by some centres, allowing a right-to-left shunt to help improve systemic output in these situations, accepting a degree of desaturation while the RV function recovers. Patients may develop pleural effusions postoperatively, particularly if they require high right atrial pressures, and indwelling chest drains may be required. Arrhythmias are the other major postoperative morbidity, either heart block related to the VSD closure or, more characteristically, His bundle tachycardia, which appears to be related to the combination of VSD closure with muscle resection in the RV. The rhythm is a narrow-complex tachycardia with dissociation of A-V conduction and does not respond to cardioversion. The rhythm will revert spontaneously with time but can cause significant haemodynamic compromise, especially if associated with restrictive physiology. Core temperature cooling can allow the rate to drop sufficiently for overdrive pacing to be effective, but supportive therapy with cooling is usually the mainstay of treatment. Amiodarone can be used cautiously, but care should be taken in younger infants as this can have an acute negative inotropic effect.

Late Outcome. The outcomes of Fallot repair are good, with 98.5 per cent survival at 30 days and 95 to 96 per cent survival at 10 and 20 years. Most patients with a trans-annular patch (60–70 per cent of all cases) will develop severe pulmonary regurgitation – this is well tolerated but leads to gradual right ventricular dilatation and diastolic dysfunction. The timing and investigation for pulmonary valve replacement are discussed in Chapter 25. Other late sequelae include residual RVOT obstruction requiring re-resection (rare) and the development of both atrial and ventricular arrhythmias, both being related to right ventricular dysfunction associated with the chronic pulmonary regurgitation. The aortic root is large in Fallot's tetralogy, but late problems with progressive root dilatation are very rare – risk factors include late age at repair and male gender.

Controversies. The role of palliation and best age for initial repair have remained areas of debate for 50 years. The general trend has been towards earlier age of repair in an attempt to avoid the need for surgical palliation. However, there remains a group of patients who present early (as neonates) with severe cyanosis or those with complex anatomy (such as Fallot combined with AVSD or anomalous LAD artery) where repair needs to be deferred until the patient is older, bigger and more stable. The Blalock-Taussig shunt remains the treatment of choice for palliation (see Chapter 4), but alternatives include placing a limiting outflow tract patch (ie leaving the VSD open but allowing a controlled amount of additional pulmonary blood flow) or placing an RVOT stent as an interventional catheter procedure. This is a bare-metal adult coronary stent (Tables 11.1 and 11.2).

Repair has the best outcomes when performed between three and nine months of age. Neonatal repair is not generally performed, as patients are not usually severely cyanotic as neonates. Timing for repair is partly guided by symptoms (degree of cyanosis), although even relatively acyanotic Fallots would usually be referred for surgery during infancy as it is well established that infant repair carries the best long-term outcomes. Avoidance of a trans-annular incision is always the aim of surgery, and RVOT obstruction

Table 11.1 Tetralogy of Fallot: Controversies

Neonatal repair verses initial palliation
Age for elective repair
Blalock-Taussig shunt versus RVOT stent or RVOT patch for palliation
Preservation of the annulus at time of repair
Creation of a competent outflow tract at repair

Table 11.2 Tetralogy of Fallot: Associations

DiGeorge syndrome, 15 per cent
DORV, 5 per cent
Right aortic arch, 15 per cent
Anomalous LAD artery, 2–5 per cent
Bilateral SVC, 10 per cent

may be preferable in the long term to the consequences of chronic severe regurgitation. Methods of preserving pulmonary competence such as the creation of monocusp of bivalved outflow tract patches and the use of static balloons to dilate the annulus at time of surgery have all been employed with variable success, and debate continues over the correct timing and indication to re-intervene on late pulmonary incompetence and right ventricular dilatation.

Further Reading

Al Habib HF, Jacobs JP, Mavroudis C et al. Contemporary patterns of management of tetralogy of Fallot: data from the STS database. *Ann Thorac Surg* 2010; **90**: 813–20.

Arenz C, Laumeier A, Lütter S et al. Is there any need for a shunt in the treatment of tetralogy of Fallot with one source of pulmonary blood flow? *Eur J Cardiothorac Surg* 2013; **44**(4): 648–54.

Hickey EJ, Veldtman G, Bradley TJ et al. Late risk of outcomes for adults with repaired tetralogy of Fallot from an inception cohort spanning four decades. *Eur J Cardiothorac Surg* 2009; **35**: 156–64.

Karl TR, Sano S, Pornviliwan S, Mee RB Tetralogy of Fallot: favorable outcome of nonneonatal transatrial, transpulmonary repair. *Ann Thorac Surg* 1992; **54**: 903–7.

Lindberg HL, Saatvedt K, Seem E, Hoel T, Birkeland S. Single-center 50 years' experience with surgical management of tetralogy of Fallot. *Eur J Cardiothorac Surg* 2011; **40**: 538–42.

Pigula FA, Khalil PN, Mayer JE, del Nido PJ, Jonas RA. Repair of tetralogy of Fallot in neonates and young infants. *Circulation* 1999; **100**: II157–61.

Robinson JD, Rathod RH, Brown DW et al. The evolving role of intraoperative balloon pulmonary valvuloplasty in valve-sparing repair of tetralogy of Fallot. *J Thorac Cardiovasc Surg* 2011; **142**(6): 1367–73.

Sarris GE, Comas JV, Tobota Z, Maruszewski B. Results of reparative surgery for tetralogy of Fallot: data from the European Association for Cardio-Thoracic Surgery Congenital Database. *Eur J Cardiothorac Surg* 2012; **42**(5): 766–74.

Walsh EP, Rockenmacher S, Keane JF et al. Late results in patients with tetralogy of Fallot repaired during infancy. *Circulation* 1988; **77**: 1062–67.

Chapter 12

Pulmonary Atresia with Major Aorto-pulmonary Collateral Arteries

David J. Barron

Introduction

Sometimes referred to as 'complex pulmonary atresia', this rare group within the spectrum of pulmonary atresia (PA)/ventricular septal defect (VSD) is defined by the additional presence of major aorto-pulmonary collateral arteries (MAPCAs) that provide multiple sources of pulmonary blood flow arising from the thoracic aorta or its branches.

Table 12.1 summarizes categorization of pulmonary atresia. The first consideration is whether there is associated VSD or not (intact septum; see Chapter 13). When a VSD is present, then this is often considered as the extreme spectrum of tetralogy of Fallot – where the outflow obstruction is so severe that it has become atretic. This is reflected in the fact that the intra-cardiac anatomy is similar to that of tetralogy with a large sub-aortic peri-membranous VSD and overriding aorta. In the majority of PA/VSD, the branch pulmonary arteries are well developed with normal branching patterns and distribution within the lungs and are supplied by the ductus arteriosus. However, approximately 20 to 40 per cent of all cases of PA/VSD are associated with MAPCAs (typically two to six vessels that arise from the thoracic aorta or the brachiocephalic artery, most commonly around the level of the carina) supplying a variable degree of the lung parenchyma. The condition is characterized by its heterogeneity and the variable relationship between the MAPCAs and the native pulmonary artery system.

Table 12.1 Classification of Pulmonary Atresia

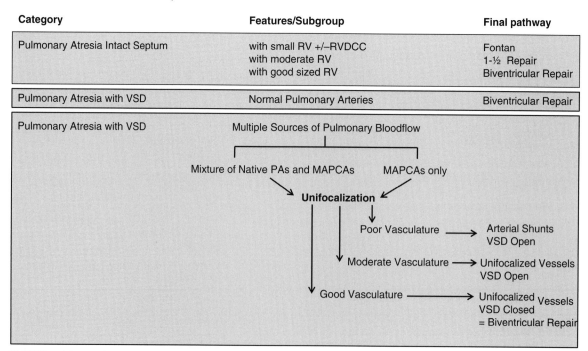

Category	Features/Subgroup	Final pathway
Pulmonary Atresia Intact Septum	with small RV +/–RVDCC with moderate RV with good sized RV	Fontan 1-½ Repair Biventricular Repair
Pulmonary Atresia with VSD	Normal Pulmonary Arteries	Biventricular Repair
Pulmonary Atresia with VSD	Multiple Sources of Pulmonary Bloodflow Mixture of Native PAs and MAPCAs ⟶ Unifocalization ⟵ MAPCAs only Poor Vasculature ⟶ Arterial Shunts / VSD Open Moderate Vasculature ⟶ Unifocalized Vessels / VSD Open Good Vasculature ⟶ Unifocalized Vessels / VSD Closed = Biventricular Repair	

RVDCC = right ventricular dependent coronary circulation.

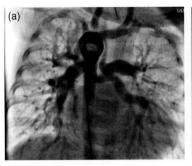
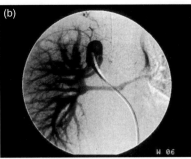
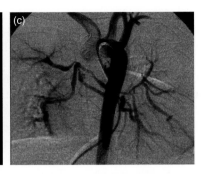

Figure 12.1 Angiographic images of three separate cases of MAPCAs. (A) Multiple large vessels supplying the entire lung parenchyma. (B) Selective angiogram of a large MAPCA showing dual supply of the right lung from both the MAPCA and the native system, feeding small native central pulmonary arteries that have the appearance of a 'seagull'. (C) Poor MAPCAs – series of small stenotic vessels with poor distribution to the lungs.

The ductus may or may not be present, but if it is present, then it will supply some component of the native system rather than a MAPCA. DiGeorge syndrome is associated with 30 per cent of cases, usually at the more severe end of the spectrum with poor-quality pulmonary vasculature.

Pulmonary blood supply can be categorized as follows:

1. Well-developed native pulmonary artery system supplying all areas of the lung. Variable MAPCAs feeding into the native system, but no areas of the lung supplied exclusively by MAPCAs.
2. Mixed distribution; under-development of native system to a variable degree with a combination of native vessels and MAPCAs supplying the lungs – some areas of the vasculature supplied exclusively by MAPCAs.
3. Complete absence of intra-pericardial pulmonary arteries. Lung supply is entirely through MAPCAs, which can be of variable size and quality.

In general, those in group 1 carry the best prognosis and those in group 3 carry the worst due to the fact that MAPCA distribution within the lung is often abnormal and underdeveloped, sometimes with tortuous and stenotic areas even within the lung tissue. However, there can still be variability even within these subgroups, and assessment of any case has to take into account the overall quality of the vasculature, which can be underdeveloped and patchy in any situation. Furthermore, the MAPCAs themselves typically run a tortuous and variable course from their origin into the lung, which can develop additional stenoses within them over time, even occluding in some cases.

Large MAPCAs can result in unprotected blood flow to areas of the lung with the risk of developing pulmonary vascular disease in these segments, whereas stenotic or small MAPCAs lead to underperfusion and potential underdevelopment of the same. Consequently, the natural history and mode of presentation of these patients are equally heterogeneous – and reflect the underlying anatomy of the pulmonary blood flow.

Presentation and Investigation. Most patients are cyanosed but relatively stable, enabling time for assessment and planning of treatment. The degree of cyanosis depends on the nature of the pulmonary blood flow, as described earlier, but severe cyanosis is unusual and is a bad prognostic sign, suggesting poorly developed vasculature. Cyanosed neonates may benefit from prostaglandin E2 if there is a ductus supplying part of the native system, but prostaglandin E2 will not have any effect on the MAPCAs themselves.

At the other end of the spectrum, patients with large MAPCAs may not be cyanosed due to such high pulmonary blood flow and are actually in congestive cardiac failure (CCF). More typically, patients lie between these two extremes and are moderately cyanosed – however, it is important to recognize that these patients are not 'safe' in that the apparently well-balanced circulation could include a mixture of some areas of the lung being over-perfused (and at risk of pulmonary vascular disease) and others under-perfused (and at risk of failing to develop).

Echocardiography is helpful to confirm the intra-cardiac anatomy and will usually identify the presence of MAPCAs arising from the aorta but cannot define the anatomy. Cardiac catheterization is essential in all cases to identify all MAPCAs and show their distribution within the lungs. Careful assessment of each injection will reveal the native system (if present) being supplied by the MAPCAs, which typically appear as a seagull-shaped image on the late phase of injection (see Figure 12.1B). MRI and CT angiography are essential adjuncts to catheterization to demonstrate the 3D relationship of the MAPCAs to the airways and the great vessels. Careful 3D reconstruction techniques are time consuming but extremely helpful for planning surgery, particularly in defining the relationship of MAPCAs to the main airways and the oesophagus (Figure 12.2).

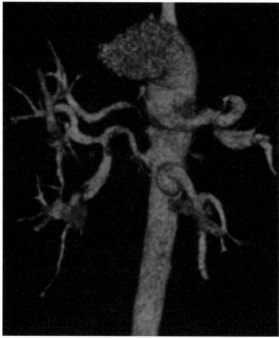

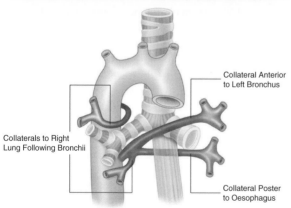

Figure 12.2 MRI reconstructive image of multiple MAPCAs and diagram demonstrating the relationship of MPACAs to the major airways and the oesophagus. (A black-and-white version of this figure will appear in some formats. For the colour version, please refer to the plate section.)

Initial Management. Most patients do not require any immediate intervention. Very cyanosed neonates may require ventilation and prostaglandin E2 while the anatomy is defined. Infants in CCF may need rapid investigation and early surgery. The focus of early management in all cases is thorough investigation to define the anatomy. When fully assessed, the aim is to plan to achieve unifocalization at between three and nine months of age.

Palliative Shunts and the Melbourne Shunt. Cyanosed patients with poor-quality vessels may be too unstable or have insufficient 'target' vessels to achieve any meaningful unifocalization. In this situation it may be necessary to simply place a systemic pulmonary shunt into the best target vessel to try to establish better oxygenation (Figure 12.3). This may stabilize the situation and allow further growth of the vessels such that subsequent unifocalization is achievable. There are some cases where there are no good-sized MAPCAs and the native intra-pericardial pulmonary arteries are present but very small. In this situation the native vessels can be connected directly into the back of the ascending aorta (or via a small Gore-Tex shunt), referred to as a 'Melbourne shunt'. This drives forward flow into the native system, and the small size of the proximal vessels should prevents any risk of over-circulation.

Unifocalization. The aim of surgery is to achieve unifocalization of as much of the pulmonary blood supply as possible. The target is to use as much of the native system as possible, but if there are areas of the lung supplied exclusively by MAPCAs, then the aim is to also recruit these vessels into the native system. Regardless of the individual anatomy, the aim is to bring as much of the pulmonary vasculature together into a single confluence and

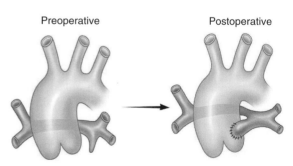

Figure 12.3 The use of a central shunt ('Melbourne shunt') to drive antegrade flow into small native central pulmonary arteries.

then drive antegrade flow into these vessels, ligating all the MAPCA origins from the aorta. This ensures controlled flow into as much of the lungs as possible, encouraging growth and development while reducing the risk of pulmonary vascular disease. Unifocalization has to be carefully planned; it can be performed entirely via median sternotomy, but access to any MAPCAs deep in the mediastinum can be difficult. It may be necessary to access the MAPCAs and mobilize them via thoracotomy before then continuing the procedure via sternotomy. This is important because being forced to go onto CPB without control of large MAPCAs can be very hazardous. Creation of a single confluence usually can be achieved using native vessels, ideally using the native PAs, laid open as a 'platform' on which to base the repair. Additional MAPCAs are disconnected from their origins and brought in to join this platform. The entire confluence is then patched open to enlarge all vessels as much as possible. Pulmonary homograft or glutaraldehyde-treated pericardium are the best tissues to use.

Closure of the VSD. The decision to close the VSD depends on the quality of the pulmonary vasculature. A useful rule of thumb is to divide each lung into 10 segments and establish how many of those segments are effectively recruited through the planned unifocalization. If more than 15 to 20 segments are recruited, closure of the VSD should be performed safely (Figure 12.4). If the pulmonary vasculature is poor (<14 segments), closing the VSD would require the whole cardiac output to be forced through these vessels, resulting in high right ventricular pressures and a risk of right ventricular failure. Thus, it is safer to leave the VSD open in these cases (or some authors prefer to perform a fenestrated VSD closure) and place a slightly smaller than full-sized RV-PA conduit to ensure there is no over-circulation. This can be a valuable option, often behaving like a mild Fallot while protecting the RV from failure and encouraging growth of the pulmonary vasculature. Subsequent closure of the VSD may still be achieved if the vasculature develops. An alternative strategy to assess pulmonary blood flow is to perfuse the unifocalized vessels with equivalent full predicted flow through the heart-lung machine and measure the pressure in the pulmonary arteries – if less than 60 per cent systemic pressure is recorded, then this should be acceptable for septation of the circulation (VSD closure). In cases where full repair is not achievable, the alternative to a limiting RV-PA conduit is to place a central shunt into the confluence, thus avoiding a ventriculotomy.

Management of each case has to be individualized to each patient and frequently requires a series of planned surgical and interventional procedures to recruit and develop the pulmonary vasculature. Serial ballooning and stenting may be necessary to overcome vessels that have stenoses within the lung, and staged shunting procedures or unifocalization may allow interim periods for growth and development of vessels (particularly those initially with poor flow).

Surgery can be demanding and time consuming, but careful control of all vessels with vascular clips enables most of the surgery to be achieved on bypass without cross-clamp. Stiff RV-PA conduits (such as Hancock or aortic homograft) are preferred so that they are able to withstand high pressures without dilating, especially if the VSD is left open.

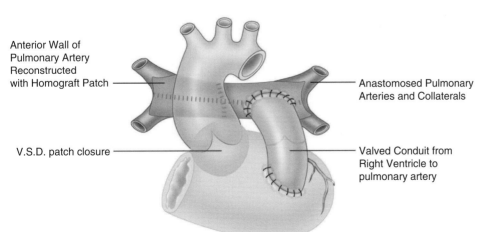

Anterior Wall of
Pulmonary Artery
Reconstructed
with Homograft Patch

Anastomosed Pulmonary
Arteries and Collaterals

V.S.D. patch closure

Valved Conduit from
Right Ventricle to
pulmonary artery

Figure 12.4 Complete unifocalization in pulmonary atresia, VSD and MAPCAs. The pulmonary arteries and MAPCAs have been unifocalized to a large confluence which is then augmented with a homograft patch. The VSD has been closed, and the repair is completed with a valved RV-PA conduit.

55

Outcomes. Overall, unifocalization can be achieved in 80 to 85 per cent of patients in most large series. There remains a group with very poor vasculature who can never achieve unifocalization and can only be palliated with systemic shunts; in-hospital mortality in this group can be 10 to 15 per cent. Operative mortality for unifocalization and repair is in the region of 4 to 8 per cent, with most patients achieving full repair (i.e. VSD closure). Numbers vary depending on institutional protocols, but the author achieved full repair in 70 per cent of this group, with a further 15 to 20 per cent achieving VSD closure at subsequent surgery. With VSD closure, a right ventricular pressure of up to 80 per cent systemic is usually acceptable (in the setting of good RV function) as the pressure tends to fall further during the early postoperative period.

Patients continue to need careful follow-up and may need serial catheter re-interventions.

Further Reading

Asija R, Koth AM, Velasquez N et al. Outcomes of children with tetralogy of Fallot, pulmonary atresia, and major aortopulmonary collaterals undergoing reconstruction of occluded pulmonary artery branches. *Ann Thorac Surg* 2016; **101**(6): 2329–34.

Davies B, Mussa S, Davies P et al. Unifocalization of major aortopulmonary collateral arteries in pulmonary atresia with ventricular septal defect is essential to achieve excellent outcomes irrespective of native pulmonary artery morphology. *J Thorac Cardiovasc Surg* 2009; **138**(6): 1269–75.

Malhotra SP, Hanley FL. Surgical management of pulmonary atresia with ventricular septal defect and major aortopulmonary collaterals: a protocol-based approach. *Semin Thorac Cardiovasc Surg Pediatr Card Surg Annu* 2009; 145–51.

Nørgaard MA, Alphonso N, Cochrane AD et al. Major aorto-pulmonary collateral arteries of patients with pulmonary atresia and ventricular septal defect are dilated bronchial arteries. *Eur J Cardiothorac Surg* 2006; **29**(5): 653–58.

Chapter 13

Pulmonary Atresia with Intact Ventricular Septum

David J. Barron

Introduction

This is an unusual condition (accounting for 5 per cent of all cases of pulmonary atresia (PA), although commoner in Eastern Asia) but one with a broad spectrum of treatment options depending on the degree of development of the right ventricle (RV). The commoner varieties of PA (i.e. PA with ventricular septal defect (VSD), tetralogy of Fallot with PA, PA with major aorto-pulmonary collateral arteries (MAPCAs)) are associated with the presence of a large VSD, which provides an outlet for the RV. However, occasionally, PA can occur in the absence of any VSD – in which case there is no outlet for the RV. This is known as 'pulmonary atresia with intact ventricular septum' (PAIVS). With no exit from the ventricular chamber, the pressure within the RV can be very high.

The consequence of this is twofold:

1. A lack of forward flow through the right ventricle can lead to varying degrees of underdevelopment or hypoplasia of the RV. This is thought to correlate with the point in fetal development at which the PA develops – the later it occurs, the better is the development of the RV.

2. The pressure within the cavity of the 'cul-de-sac' of the RV can become very high, leading to myocardial hypertrophy, endocardial damage and the creation of fistulous communications between the (high-pressure) RV cavity and the coronary arterial circulation. If these fistulae become well developed, then flow into the coronary circulation becomes retrograde from the right ventricular cavity into (usually) the right coronary system. In severe cases, the consequence is that the coronary circulation becomes dependent on this retrograde flow driven by high right ventricular pressure (so-called right ventricular-dependent coronary circulation), and the fistulous flow creates a dilated right coronary system. This creates a fragile coronary circulation at risk of coronary steal, typically in situations of low aortic diastolic pressure (Figure 13.1).

The key to management and the ultimate destination in this condition is based on assessment of the RV size. The normal RV is described as being 'tripartite', consisting of an inlet portion, an outlet portion and an apical trabecular portion. Assessing the volume of the right ventricular cavity in a neonate can be very difficult in view of its multiple thick trabeculations and its asymmetrical shape, and echocardiographic assessment of right ventricular volume is notoriously unreliable. Thus, the tricuspid valve dimension is usually used as a surrogate marker of right ventricular size and based on the Z-score of the predicted size according to body surface area (BSA). Table 13.1 summarizes the predictive outcome for the RV in the setting of PAIVS based on tricuspid valve size. RVs that are 'bipartite' (i.e. no apical trabecular portion) are very rarely likely to be suitable for biventricular repair.

Diagnosis and Presentation

Patients present as newborns with cyanosis, and survival is duct dependent. Patients with a patent ductus may remain stable but will have varying degree of cyanosis, but if presentation is at the time of duct closure, then the baby may present with circulatory collapse and need resuscitation and ventilation. All patients need prostaglandin E2 infusion.

The mainstay of diagnosis is with echocardiography, and other imaging modalities are not usually required. MRI or CT may be indicated if there is concern about the branch pulmonary artery anatomy or size. Echo will confirm the diagnosis and also define the structure and size of the RV (atrial septum above, with particular focus on tricuspid valve (TV) size) as well as the presence of any coronary fistulae.

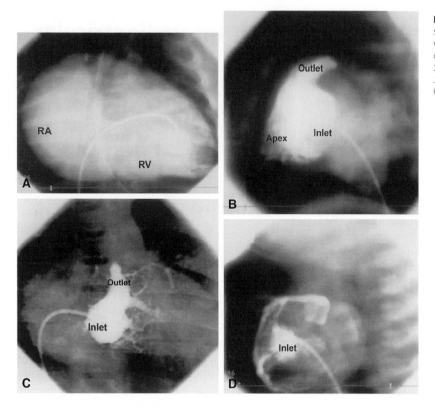

Figure 13.1 Angiographic image showing small right ventricular cavity with right ventricular-dependent coronary circulation.
Source: From Daubeney PEF et al. Journal American College of Cardiology. 2002, 15:39(10):1670–9

Table 13.1 Predictive Outcome for the RV in the Setting of PAIVS Based on Tricuspid Valve Size

Z-score of tricuspid valve	Composition of RV	Likely destination
Larger than −2	Tripartite	Biventricular repair
−2 to −5	Tripartite ± bipartite	1½-Type repair
Smaller than −5	Bipartite	Univentricular repair (Fontan pathway)

Neonatal Management

Initial management in all cases is to secure adequate pulmonary blood flow. However, the aim of treatment is also to decompress the high-pressure right ventricular cavity in all cases, except those where the RV is so small that it is unlikely to be of any use (Z-score < −5).

1. Typically there is membranous atresia of the pulmonary valve with an adequate-sized pulmonary annulus that can be crossed in the catheterization laboratory with either a plain wire or a radio-frequency wire and then ballooned. The procedure carries a risk of perforating the heart, which may need emergency surgical rescue, but is generally a safe procedure, keeping the duct open on a prostaglandin infusion.

2. If radio-frequency perforation fails or is not felt to be achievable, then the valve can be opened surgically, often placing a small trans-annular patch to ensure an adequate-sized outflow tract. The patent ductus can be snared during the procedure and then released after completion to provide additional pulmonary blood flow if necessary.

Patients with large coronary fistulae should *not* undergo decompression of the RV as this may lead to sudden coronary steal and ischaemia. The presence of coronary fistulae is a recognized risk factor for survival after Blalock-Taussig (BT) shunt, related to the fact that the low diastolic pressure in the setting of such a shunt increases the risk of coronary steal phenomena.

3. The RV tends to remain stiff and restrictive, even in the best of cases with well-developed right

ventricular size. Take into account that the RV tends to shrink in volume once the high pressure has been released and that pulmonary vascular resistance is still high in the newborn – and the consequence is that these patients will almost always need some additional source of pulmonary blood flow for at least the short term. The simplest thing is to keep the duct open on a prostaglandin infusion, but if the duct becomes unreliable or if the patient remains duct dependent, then either a BT shunt or ductal stenting will be required. Patients will tend to shunt right to left across the ASD, but saturations in the 1970s and 1980s are perfectly safe, and in patients with a good-sized RV, the saturations may gradually rise over the following few days as the pulmonary vascular resistance (PVR) drops and the RV becomes less restrictive. Inhaled nitric oxide (iNO) can be used in unstable patients, and milrinone or phosphodiesterase inhibitors may help reduce right ventricular stiffness.

Subsequent Management

Neonatal intervention should stabilize the circulation, although it may be several years before a final decision can be made. The size and volume of the RV will dictate decision making.

1. A very small RV with a TV Z-score of less than −5 will normally have been left with imperforate valve and have been stabilized with a BT shunt or ductal stent. These patients will progress down a Fontan pathway, with a bidirectional Glenn shunt being the next stage. It is important to ensure that the atrial septum is unrestrictive.

2. Tripartite RV with TV Z-score greater than −2 should achieve biventricular repair. Often this is self-evident, and after initial opening of the outflow tract (either with balloon or surgery), biventricular repair has been achieved. Some cases may have required a BT shunt as a neonate in the setting of a stiff ventricle, but as diastolic function improves, the BT shunt can be ligated and the atrial septum closed. Echo and catheter findings will direct decision making, and any residual stenosis in the outflow tract may need to be addressed to achieve complete repair. Most patients will have significant pulmonary regurgitation, which is usually well tolerated. Pulmonary valve replacement may be necessary later in life along the same criteria as in repaired tetralogy of Fallot.

3. Borderline cases (TV Z-score −2 to −5), where the RV is felt to be too small to support the circulation unaided, can undergo a bidirectional Glenn shunt with either closing the atrial septum or leaving a small ASD. This is known as the '1½-type repair', where the RV is essentially handling only the inferior vena cava (IVC) return and is a valuable option in this small group of truly borderline cases. This provides good quality of life with normal oxygen saturations, although exercise capability is not usually as good as in full biventricular repair.

The 'right ventricular overhaul' operation is an additional consideration in borderline RVs where right ventricular volume is maximized by dividing and resecting muscle bundles in the RV and ensuring that tricuspid leaflets are fully opened and that the outflow tract is unrestrictive. This can help maximize the right ventricular volume but is only applicable to a small number of borderline cases, particularly where the apical portion of the RV is very muscle bound. In selected patients, the effective right ventricular volume can be increased, but the Z-score of the TV does not change or 'grow'.

Coronary artery fistulae are generally left untreated. They are usually only seen in the very small RVs in which there is no question of attempting biventricular or even 1½-type repair. Some authors have suggested ligation of large fistulae that are visible on the epicardial surface of the heart, but this has rarely been attempted.

Outcomes

The greatest risk is in the first six months of life. Patients who survive beyond this have an excellent prognosis. Patients with right ventricular-dependent coronary circulation (RVDCC) are those at greatest risk, and six-month survival is 70 per cent.

The spectrum of disease differs across the globe, but in Western countries, around 30 to 35 per cent of all cases are expected to achieve biventricular repair, and a further 5 per cent have a 1½-type circulation.

Duct-dependent neonates with PA/IVS are among the highest risk groups of neonates, especially those requiring BT shunts. The small group of PA/IVS patients who have a RV-dependent coronary circulation remain at slightly higher risk even after Fontan completion.

Further Reading

Bryant R 3rd, Nowicki ER, Mee RB et al. Success and limitations of right ventricular sinus myectomy for pulmonary atresia with intact ventricular septum *J Thorac Cardiovasc Surg* 2008; **136**(3): 735–42.

Daubeney PE, Wang D, Delany DJ et al. Pulmonary atresia with intact ventricular septum: predictors of early and medium-term outcome in a population-based study. *J Thorac Cardiovasc Surg* 2005; **130**: 1071.

Giglia TM, Jenkins KJ, Matitiau A et al. Influence of right heart size on outcome in pulmonary atresia with intact ventricular septum. *Circulation* 1993; **88**: 2248–56.

Guleserian KJ, Armsby LB, Thiagarajan RR, del Nido PJ, Mayer JE Jr. Natural history of pulmonary atresia with intact ventricular septum and right-ventricle-dependent coronary circulation managed by the single-ventricle approach. *Ann Thorac Surg* 2006; **81**(6): 2250–57.

Chapter 14

Aortic Valve Disease and Left Outflow Tract Obstruction

David J. Barron

Introduction

Congenital abnormalities of the left outflow tract can be categorized into sub-valvar, valvar and supra-valvar components. Hypoplasia of the whole left outflow tract is usually part of the spectrum of hypoplastic left heart syndrome (see Chapter 20) and should be managed accordingly, but this chapter considers left ventricular outflow tract (LVOT) problems in the setting of an otherwise adequate-sized left ventricle.

Sub-Aortic Stenosis. The commonest form of sub-aortic stenosis is a circumferential fibrous membrane developing immediately beneath the aortic valve leaflets (Figure 14.1). It is usually well defined but can extend onto the underside of the leaflets and along the ventricular septum. The aetiology may be due to the initial presence of a small, restrictive sub-aortic ventricular septal defect (VSD) that is closed by fibrous tissue generated by the turbulent flow. The build-up of fibrous tissue in the outflow tract then generates more turbulence, and there is further accumulation, creating a circumferential ridge of tissue. The lesion most commonly occurs in isolation but can be seen in association with atrio-ventricular septal defect (AVSD). The dimensions and structure of the aortic valve are usually normal, but if the membrane is extending onto the valve leaflets, they can become tethered with progressive aortic regurgitation. There may be a muscular component to the obstruction, partly due to the compensatory hypertrophy of the left ventricle (LV) in response to the stenosis. Purely muscular sub-aortic stenosis is usually an acquired lesion related to asymmetrical septal hypertrophy as part of hypertrophic obstructive cardiomyopathy (HOCM). Longer, tubular stenosis of the LVOT is rare and most likely seen in the setting of repaired AVSD (with its 'goose-necked' LVOT, which predisposes to stenosis; see Chapter 10) or repaired double-outlet right ventricle (DORV) or transposition of the great arteries (TGA)/VSD, where the VSD has been

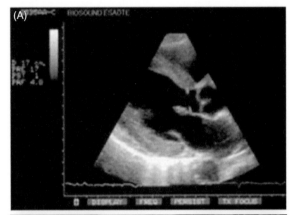

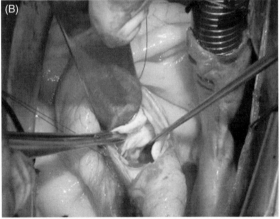

Figure 14.1 Echo image of (A) discrete sub-aortic membrane and (B) operative view through the aortic valve.
Source: From Kratiochvil F et al. Cor et Vasa Volume 59, Issue 5, October 2017, Pages e436–e440.
(A black-and-white version of this figure will appear in some formats. For the colour version, please refer to the plate section.)

closed with a patch that commits the LV through to the displaced aorta.

Investigation and Management. Trans-thoracic echo will provide all the necessary information in the majority of cases, but occasionally trans-oesophageal echo (TOE) or even MRI is helpful in more complex tunnel-like stenoses. It is important to establish how close any membrane is to the valve and whether or not the leaflets are tethered. A peak gradient of more than 50 mmHg is generally regarded as an indication for surgery. Stenosis is not amenable to ballooning or stenting as it is a fixed fibro-muscular obstruction. The only situation where non-surgical treatment is an option is in the rare situation of asymmetrical septal hypertrophy in HOCM where radio-frequency muscle ablation has been attempted, as well as selective alcohol injection into the first septal perforator branch of the left anterior descending (LAD) coronary artery. However, these techniques require highly specialized interventional cardiologists and are usually reserved for adults or older adolescents.

Surgery for isolated sub-aortic stenosis is performed through a standard aortotomy, working through the aortic valve (Figure 14.1B). The fibrous shelf is incised where it meets the septal muscle underneath the commissure of the left and right coronary cusps. The membrane can then be peeled away from the muscle. Care should be taken to peel away any extensions of the membrane onto the underside of the valve cusps. If possible, a wedge resection of septal muscle is also performed (again, working beneath the commissure between the left and right coronary cusps so as to be distant from the bundle) to maximize the area beneath the aortic valve and so reduce the risk of recurrence. The leaflets must be carefully checked at the end of the procedure to ensure that they have not been injured.

More complex tunnel obstruction may have a fibrous component that can be resected in a similar way together with any hypertrophied muscle bulging into the outflow tract – especially if there has been previous surgery with subsequent fibrous reaction. Long-length tubular obstruction in the setting of an adequate-sized aortic valve is exceedingly rare. A Konno procedure can be considered in this situation: a transverse incision is made in the infundibulum of the right ventricle, and the aorta is opened through a standard incision (Figure 14.2). An instrument is then passed through the aortic valve and pushed through the thickened septal muscle to appear on the right ventricular side. The intervening muscle is then cored out to create a large VSD under the aortic valve, and the defect repaired with a patch placed on the right ventricular side of the septum. This is an unusual and difficult procedure, carrying significant risk of heart block and ventricular dysfunction. More commonly,

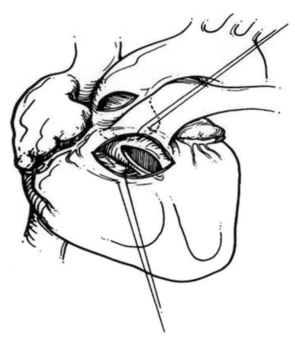

Figure 14.2 Konno procedure for LVOT stenosis.
Source: From Roughneen PT et al. Annals of Thoracic Surgery Volume 65, Issue 5, May 1998, Pages 1368–1376.

the aortic valve is also small, and the septum can be opened in combination with excising the aortic valve, splitting the aortic annulus and then combining this with a Ross procedure (see below and Figure 14.3), such as the 'Ross-Konno' procedure or with patch enlargement and placement of a prosthetic aortic valve (Konno-Rastan).

In the setting of functionally univentricular circulations, complex sub-aortic stenosis can sometimes be managed by creating a 'double outlet' to the heart and joining the pulmonary and aortic roots together in what is called the 'Damus-Kaye-Stansel (DKS) procedure' (Figure 14.4). This is only possible where there is a normally developed pulmonary valve and root and is typically seen in the setting of double-inlet left ventricle (DILV), where the aorta arises from a vestigial right ventricle (see Chapter 4).

Supra-aortic Stenosis. This is rare and usually occurs in isolation and in the setting of a normal tri-leaflet aortic valve of normal dimension. The lesion has a characteristic 'hourglass' deformity immediately above (sometime involving) the sino-tubular junction and can be very pronounced (Figure 14.5). It is most commonly associated with Williams syndrome, a deletion of part of the long arm of chromosome 7

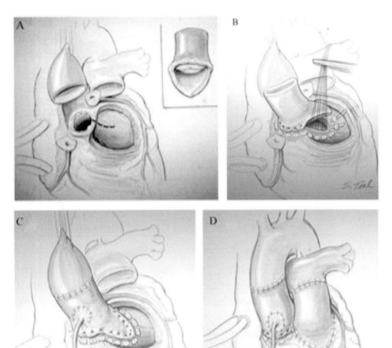

Figure 14.3 Ross-Konno procedure: note that the pulmonary autograft is harvested with a 'skirt' of RV muscle attached which can be used to augment the defect created in the left outflow tract in performing the Konno incision.
Source: From Brown JW et al. Annals of Thoracic Surgery Volume 82, Issue 4, October 2006, Pages 1301–1306.

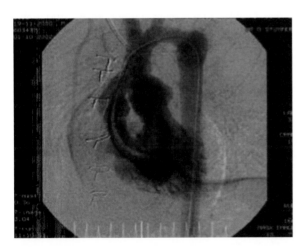

Figure 14.4 Damus-Kaye-Stansel procedure showing the aorta and main pulmonary artery joined together. Note that the patient previously underwent arch repair with a subclavian flap technique.

which is characterized by 'elfin-like' facial features, mild to moderate developmental delay and an overly sociable personality. Supra-aortic stenosis is the commonest cardiac lesion, but there may also be multiple stenoses in the central and branch pulmonary arteries, the latter of which tend to regress with age. Williams accounts for about 60 to 70 per cent of all cases of supra-aortic stenosis. The aortic wall is very thickened, contributing to the stenosis, and there can be associated origin stenosis of head and neck vessels and tubular narrowing of the transverse arch.

Investigation and Management. Trans-thoracic echo confirms the diagnosis, but CT angiography and cardiac catheter are also required to confirm the relationship of the coronary arteries to the narrowing and to provide imaging of the aortic arch, head and neck vessels and branch pulmonary arteries, which can also be involved.

There is no place for ballooning or stenting of the supra-aortic region as it is too close to the valve and coronary arteries. Surgery is the definite treatment, and repair can be achieved in a variety of ways: the ascending aorta is incised longitudinally across the region of narrowing to split the thickened ring into the non-

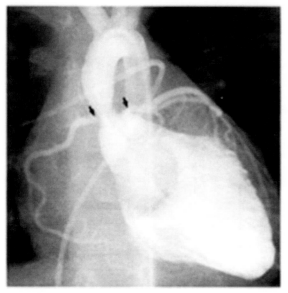

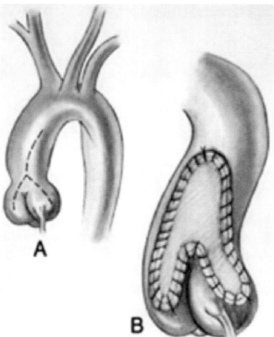

Figure 14.5 Angiographic image of supra-aortic stenosis and diagram showing Y-patch technique of repair.
Source: From Stamm C et al. Journal of Thoracic and Cardiovascular Surgery Volume 118, Issue 5, November 1999, Pages 874–88.

coronary sinus and then patch repaired (single-patch technique). More commonly, a Y-shaped incision is made, crossing the narrowed ridge at two points into the non-coronary and right coronary cusps and repaired with a Y-shaped patch (Y-shaped patch technique; Figure 14.5). Alternatively, the aorta is transected above the narrowing, and three separate patches are placed into the each sinus; this is known as the 'Brom technique'.

All techniques have been used with success, but the Y-shaped patch and Brom techniques have the best long-term outcomes with equally good freedom from re-stenosis (90 per cent at 10 years) and an operative mortality of 2 to 3 per cent. Significant branch pulmonary artery narrowing may also be addressed at the same procedure, but these narrowings tend to have a more benign natural history and can be managed more conservatively if right ventricular pressures are not significantly raised.

Aortic Valve Disease. The commonest congenital abnormality is the bicuspid aortic valve, which is present in up to 2 per cent of the population. The majority of cases are functionally normal and may never reach clinical significance or present only in adulthood – hence are not always strictly categorized as 'congenital' heart disease. Variable degrees and severity of leaflet dysplasia are seen, most commonly in the setting of a tri-leaflet valve, but in more severe cases, it can be difficult to identify any normal valve structure, with the valve being no more than a mass of thickened and irregular dysplastic tissue and no identifiable commissures. The predominant lesion is stenosis, but there can be associated regurgitation of the valve. Presentation depends on the severity of stenosis and can be at birth in the most severe cases. Life-threatening aortic stenosis at birth is referred to as 'critical aortic stenosis', where there is inadequate cardiac output across the LVOT, and there is a duct-dependent circulation – this can be associated with global underdevelopment of the left ventricle (LV) and fall into the spectrum of 'borderline LV' and even 'hypoplastic left heart syndrome' (see Chapter 20). In childhood, aortic valve stenosis can be associated with a slightly small aortic annulus and sub-valvar area despite a good-sized left ventricle, and this needs to be taken into account in surgical management. Isolated aortic regurgitation in congenital heart disease is rare but can be seen secondary to the dilated root of connective tissue disease such as Marfan syndrome or Loewys-Dietz syndrome. Other causes of regurgitation are secondary to rheumatic fever (rare in developed countries and usually a combination of regurgitation and stenosis) or endocarditis. Finally, regurgitation can be associated with the presence of a sub-aortic VSD of doubly committed orientation, in which the aortic valve cusp (usually the right coronary cusp) is prolapsing into the defect, becoming stretched, and may even become sealed into the defect, effectively closing the VSD.

Investigation and Management. Critical aortic stenosis presents at birth and requires stabilization with prostaglandin E2 and may need ventilation and inotropic support. However, outside the neonatal period, moderate and even severe aortic valve disease is usually well tolerated, and children are frequently asymptomatic. Trans-thoracic echo will establish the diagnosis in all cases and provide information on left ventricular function and dimensions, as well as assessment of associated lesions. In older children, trans-oesophageal echo (TOE) may also give more detailed imaging of the valve leaflets and sub-valvar area. On Doppler flow, a peak velocity of more than 50 mmHg is generally regarded as an indication for intervention even in symptomless children (note that in the setting of impaired ventricular function the degree of stenosis by Doppler can be underestimated). Aortic regurgitation can be more difficult to quantify, although the width and length of the regurgitant jet on echo can be helpful. Evidence of reversed diastolic flow in the aortic arch and wide pulse pressure suggests at least moderate regurgitation. In symptomless children, monitoring left ventricular dimensions can be helpful, referring to standard nomograms of LVEDD and LVESD according to body surface area (BSA). Deviation by +2 Z-scores or more is generally an indication for surgery. 3D echo can help to characterize the leaflet abnormalities and motion.

ECG is very important and will provide evidence of left ventricular hypertrophy (LVH) and, in severe case, of left ventricular strain. 3D imaging such as CT angiography or MRI can be used if there is concern over the aortic arch, and it is also necessary in supra-aortic stenosis to define the anatomy and to exclude associated stenoses on other arteries (especially the head and neck origins and renal arteries) and the pulmonary tree. MRI can also be helpful in quantifying regurgitation as it can be used to calculate a regurgitant fraction. CT/MRI is also essential in connective tissue disease to identify abnormalities in the thoracic and abdominal aorta. Cardiac catheterization is not usually necessary unless there is need to define coronary anatomy in supra-aortic stenosis or if the echo assessment of severity is equivocal, and a direct pressure gradient is needed to define the degree of stenosis. A peak pressure gradient of more

than 50 to 60 mmHg on echo is regarded as an indication for intervention, but decisions have to take into account the age of the patient and associated lesions. The derived gradient may be deceptively low in the presence of impaired ventricular function, and the threshold for intervention will be less – similarly, mixed stenosis with moderate or greater regurgitation will also merit intervention.

Surgical Options

Aortic Valvotomy and Repair. Preservation of the native aortic valve is the first aim of treatment. Fused commissures can be opened back to the aortic wall and the leaflets thinned out, resecting thickened nodules and false raphes to improve leaflet mobility. Care has to be taken to ensure that each leaflet is still adequately supported, and if a commissure has to be taken down or is unsupported, then a 'butterfly patch' can be sewn to the aortic wall and then attached to each neighbouring leaflet to provide support. There is no ideal material for leaflet reconstruction, but best results have been achieved with glutaraldehyde-preserved autologous pericardium with increasing interest in decellularized xenograft patches. The outcomes of aortic valvotomy/repair depend on the underlying condition of the ventricle and the urgency of presentation. In neonates with critical aortic stenosis, the operative mortality is 5 to 15 per cent, and it may be necessary to allow the patent ductus arteriosus (PDA) to reopen at the end of the procedure and even to place bilateral PA bands to allow the RV to help support the systemic circulation. In non-duct-dependent infants and older children, the operative risk is in the region of 1 per cent.

Aortic Valve Repair/Reconstruction. Valve repair techniques for the aortic valve, predominantly in the setting of regurgitation, have gained increasing interest over the past 10 years. Most success has been achieved where the valve leaflets are relatively normal and regurgitation is secondary to a dilated annulus or to a dilated sino-tubular junction (STJ) causing displacement of the commissures. Restoration of normal annular dimension with an external collar around the root, sub-commissural annuloplasties and stabilization of the STJ are the primary techniques, but most are only suitable in older children, in whom there is no longer any need to allow for growth. Many cases of connective tissue disease fall into this category, where a valve-sparing root procedure, most commonly with an implantation technique and a Valsalva graft, not only abolishes the regurgitation but also replaces the abnormal ascending aorta to prevent the risk of subsequent dilation, rupture or dissection. In the elective setting, the risks of a valve-sparing root are less than 1 per cent, with reduction in aortic regurgitation in 85 to 90 per cent of patients.

Complete three-leaflet reconstruction of the aortic valve has been attempted in the past, but most cases still required subsequent replacement. More recently, the Ozakie technique using sized templates to create each leaflet has met with improved results in older children. Early results are very good, but concerns remain over there being no ideal material and early failure of the valve due to thickening and stiffening of the xenograft or glutaraldehyde-preserved tissue.

Ross Procedure (Pulmonary Autograft). This aortic valve replacement technique involves taking the patient's own pulmonary valve (as a root) and re-implanting it into the aortic position, usually as a complete root. This has the advantage of using the patient's autologous and living tissue as a valve replacement – with the unique advantage of a valve replacement that will 'grow' with the patient. The technique can be used at any age (even neonate) and has extremely good haemodynamics as it retains much of the shape and elasticity of a native aortic root. The pulmonary valve has to be replaced – ideally with a pulmonary homograft (but xenograft conduits can be used). This the first-choice aortic valve replacement in any growing child and has the added flexibility that the outflow tract can also be enlarged by splitting the aortic annulus and opening the ventricular septum (Ross-Konno; Figure 14.3) in children with a small LVOT. The Ross procedure is complex, and care has be taken in harvesting the autograft to avoid the first septal branch of the left coronary artery and, in symmetrical implantation of the autograft, to ensure a competent valve. Operative outcomes are excellent, with an operative risk of 1 to 2 per cent in the elective setting. Risk is higher in neonates, in whom there may be associated left ventricular dysfunction and associated lesions. The greatest concern with the Ross procedure is mid- to long-term dilatation of the autograft leading to aortic regurgitation and even root aneurysm. Techniques to reinforce the autograft at the time of insertion may reduce this risk, but these have to allow some ability for growth in smaller children. Reoperation for autograft dilation

is around 10 per cent at 15 years, although many can be treated with a valve-sparing root procedure.

Non-Ross Aortic Valve Replacement. In non-repairable valves, the choice of valve replacement is mainly dictated by size. Aortic homografts are the most versatile choice and can be a useful alternative if Ross is not possible (such as with an abnormal pulmonary valve). They are usually implanted as a full root replacement but can but implanted freehand as a sub-coronary valve in older children. Homografts will calcify and degenerate in the great majority of cases but can be a valuable interim solution until the child is old enough for a prosthetic valve.

In older children who can accommodate a standard prosthetic valve the choice between a mechanical and bioprosthetic valve is much as for an adult. Both can be safely used, and decision is a balance between the risks of anticoagulation and the early degeneration of bioprosthetic valves in young adults. Although the risks of bleeding and thromboembolism are small for AVR in young people (0.8% per year) this is still a significant cumulative risk over a lifetime and there are many lifestyle issues that need to be considered in making these choices.

Further Reading

Alsoufi B, Al-Halees Z, Manlhiot C et al. Mechanical valves versus the Ross procedure for aortic valve replacement in children: propensity-adjusted comparison of long-term outcomes *J Thorac Cardiovasc Surg* 2009; **137**: 362–70.

Brown JW, Ruzmetov M, Vijay P, Rodefeld MD, Turrentine MW. The Ross-Konno procedure in children: outcomes, autograft and allograft function, and reoperations. *Ann Thorac Surg* 2006; **82**(4): 1301–6.

Kramer P, Absi D, Hetzer R et al. Outcome of surgical correction of congenital supravalvular aortic stenosis with two- and three-sinus reconstruction techniques. *Ann Thorac Surg* 2014; **97**(2): 634–40.

Lo Rito M, Davies B, Brawn WJ et al. Comparison of the Ross/Ross-Konno aortic root in children before and after the age of 18 months. *Eur J Cardiothorac Surg* 2014; **46**(3): 450–57.

Ozaki S, Kawase I, Yamashita H et al. Aortic valve reconstruction using autologous pericardium for patients aged less than 60 years. *Thorac Cardiovasc Surg* 2014; **148**(3): 934–38.

Vricella LA, Cameron DE. Valve-sparing aortic root replacement in pediatric patients: lessons learned over two decades. *Semin Thorac Cardiovasc Surg Pediatr Card Surg Annu* 2017; **20**: 56.

Chapter 15

Tricuspid Valve Abnormalities in Congenital Heart Disease

David J. Barron

Introduction

It is difficult to separate discussion of the tricuspid valve (TV) from that of the right ventricle (RV) because abnormalities of TV function are usually associated, or even caused by, degrees of right ventricular dysfunction. In the normal circulation, the low pressure in the RV allows the TV to function under low stress with low afterload and so even moderate degrees of TV dysfunction are generally well tolerated. In considering the abnormalities of the TV, it is best to consider them under the following four headings:

1. The TV in the setting of biventricular circulation
2. The TV in the systemic RV
3. The TV in the functionally univentricular circulation
4. Ebstein's anomaly of the TV

Tricuspid Valve in Biventricular Circulation

Congenital isolated abnormalities of the TV are rare. Tricuspid stenosis is more commonly a surrogate marker of a small RV and so is rather a degree of 'hypoplasia' of the valve rather than valvular narrowing. Tricuspid regurgitation (TR) is commoner, but the majority is functional regurgitation secondary to volume overload of the RV (such as with large atrial septal defects (ASDs) or due to chronic pulmonary regurgitation after repair of Fallot's tetralogy) or right ventricular strain (such as with pulmonary stenosis with no VSD). Primary valvar causes of TR include isolated dysplasia of the leaflets, leaflet clefts (most commonly in the anterior leaflet) and flail/elongated chordae. Acquired TR is commoner than primary valve dysplasia and is most likely to be due to damage or tethering of the septal leaflet after VSD (or Fallot) repair or damage to the valve leaflet during an interventional catheter procedure or secondary to an endocardial pacing wire across the valve (see Table 15.1).

Clinical Presentation and Investigation. Hypoplasia of the TV and small/borderline RV is dealt with in Chapter 13; however, isolated stenosis of the TV can cause liver engorgement and exercise intolerance in severe cases. If there is a small ASD, then there may be right-to-left shunting causing a degree of cyanosis – this may be the presenting feature. TR in the absence of other lesions is usually very well tolerated, especially in childhood, and rarely causes any symptoms. Trans-thoracic echocardiography is the mainstay of investigation and gives excellent anatomical and functional assessment of the valve. The Carpentier principles of valve assessment should be applied, looking at annular dilatation, leaflet motion and sub-valvar apparatus in turn. Secondary causes of regurgitation are very common, and care should be taken to look for any associated lesions or cause for right ventricular dysfunction. 3D echo can be helpful in understanding the mechanism of regurgitation, but investigation modalities other than echo are rarely

Table 15.1 Causes of Tricuspid Regurgitation in Congenital Heart Disease

1. **Secondary to dilatation:**

   Volume overload of RV – ASDs or chronic PR after Fallot repair
   Right ventricular strain due to high afterload: pulmonary stenosis, conduit degeneration or out-growth

2. **Congenital valvar abnormalities;**

   Ebstein's anomaly
   Leaflet cleft
   Elongated or ruptured chordate
   Dysplasia of leaflets

3. **Iatrogenic/postoperative/acquired:**

   Tethering of septal leaflet after VSD closure
   Injury during previous catheter intervention
   Injury/fibrosis related to an endocardial pacing wire
   Endocarditis

4. **The tricuspid valve in the systemic circulation:**

   Secondary to right ventricular dysfunction and dilatation
   Secondary to displacement of the interventricular septum under pressure load

needed. In cases of secondary TR, the investigations will be guided by the nature of the underlying lesions (e.g. ASD may need MRI and cardiac catheter to assess right ventricular volume and Qp:Qs).

Surgical Management. In the rare cases of isolated valvar stenosis with a normal-sized annulus, surgical commissurotomy may be possible, but thickened and dysplastic stenosed valves may require replacement. Regurgitant valves are generally very amenable to repair because the low-pressure environment of the right-sided circulation and compliance of the RV will provide a good setting to accommodate durable repair. Additionally, the aetiology of regurgitation is usually secondary – and surgery will usually involve concomitant repair/correction of the primary problem, which then optimizes the chance for successful repair.

Annuloplasty. Circumferential annuloplasty using a double-layered suture (De Vega annuloplasty) is the most commonly used technique for symmetrical dilatation of the TV annulus. The sutures follow the true annulus at the hinge points of the valve and avoid the septal component of the annulus in the triangle of Koch to avoid risking injury to the A-V node and bundle. Sutures are reinforced with soft pledgets and tied down with a dilator passed through the valve orifice of a size equivalent to the predicted size for the patient's weight/body surface area (BSA) (Figure 15.1A). Partial annuloplasties for more asymmetrical valves or correcting more localized jets of regurgitation include commissural annuloplasties or the Kaye annuloplasty, which is predominantly based on the inferior leaflet (Figure 15.1B). Choice depends on the symmetry of the valve and is guided by the echo assessment. Adolescents or adults with no need to accommodate for growth could have an annuloplasty ring to provide a sturdier support for the valve. However, since most patients are younger and are also having the primary lesion addressed, a fixed ring is not always necessary. There is some evidence that older adult patients (>30 years) with severe regurgitation will have a more durable result with a ring rather than simple annuloplasty suture.

Leaflet Repair. True clefts are unusual but most commonly seen in the anterior leaflet. These can be closed primarily and are often combined with a simple annuloplasty. Localized regurgitation due

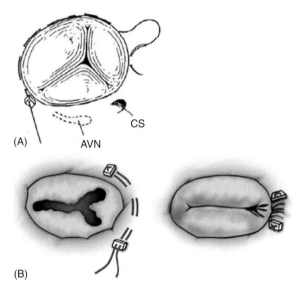

Figure 15.1 (A) De-Vega annuloplasty. (B) Partial annuloplasty. *Source*: Seminars in Thoracic and Cardiovascular Surgery: Pediatric Cardiac Surgery Annual Volume 15, Issue 1, 2012, Pages 61–68, Tsang V et al. (a) and Volume 14, Issue 1, 2011, Pages 75–84, Honjo O et al. (b).

to natural crenulations in the leaflets has been described, and closing these areas together in a similar fashion can be effective.

Prolapse. Localized areas of prolapse can be managed by fixing the region to the neighbouring leaflet tissue, combined with local annuloplasty – again due to the forgiving nature of the low-pressured RV. Ruptured or absent chordae can be replaced with artificial chords (Gore-Tex) to fix the height of the leaflet. This can be difficult in younger children, and edge-to-edge apposition of the prolapsed segment to its natural opposite leaflet (Alfieri stitch) is a valuable technique if more standard repair cannot be achieved. Again, the low-pressure environment of the RV allows for good durability of the Alfieri technique. Localized triangular or quadrangular resections of leaflets (popular in adult mitral valve repair) are not generally necessary.

Sub-valvar Correction. Chordal shortening of elongated chords is possible but ideally should be accompanied by placement of artificial chords to help fix the chordal length. Wide separation of the papillary muscles, usually partly due to dilatation of the RV, can be partially corrected by advancing the anterior papillary muscle to the ventricular septum with a double-armed pledgetted suture. This is usually combined with some degree of annuloplasty to further support the valve.

The Tricuspid Valve in the Systemic Circulation

Rarely, the TV can be in the systemic circulation. This is most commonly in the setting of congenitally corrected transposition (see Chapter 18) but is also seen in older patients with d-type transposition of the great arteries (d-TGA) who had been palliated with an atrial switch (Senning or Mustard) in the previous era. In this situation, the TV itself is usually structurally normal, but the systemic pressure in the RV leads to a more globular-shaped ventricle with subsequent bowing of the ventricular septum – and since the TV has chordal attachment to the septum, this has the effect of pulling the leaflets apart, usually with additional strain and dilatation on the tricuspid annulus. The result is TR, and there is then a complex and ongoing interaction between the TR and progressive dilatation and dysfunction of the systemic RV that leads to a vicious cycle of further TR and further right ventricular dysfunction.

Clinical Presentation and Investigation. Physiologically, this will present as for mitral regurgitation in the normally connected circulation, with failure to thrive, tachypnoea and decreased exercise tolerance, depending on the age of the child. Moderate degrees of regurgitation are often well tolerated in children and produce few symptoms, but severe cases develop signs of congestive cardiac failure. Echocardiography will confirm the diagnosis, and careful assessment of the associated right ventricular dysfunction is essential. MRI can be helpful, especially in older children and adults, to objectively measure right ventricular ejection fraction.

Surgical Management. Surgical management is very different to that above. As discussed in Chapter 4, pulmonary artery (PA) banding can have a dramatic effect on the degree of TR in many cases – the mechanism being that the band pressurizes the sub-pulmonary ventricle and so splints the ventricular septum, straightening it up and pushing it back towards the RV (Figure 15.2). This can help to stabilize the TV and reduce regurgitation. However, this is not usually a long-term solution and is frequently part of a planned and staged process towards ultimate double switch. Indeed, many would argue that the best way to treat TR in congenitally corrected transposition of the great arteries (ccTGA) is simply to get the tricuspid valve out of the systemic circulation. Conversely, isolated repair of the TV in this setting has extremely disappointing results with almost universal recurrence of regurgitation within five years – although performing repair with concurrent PA banding may produce better results (data are difficult to interpret because most of these patients are on track for planned double switch). Older patients, in

Pre- Banding: severe TR

Post- Banding: septum splinted reduction in TR

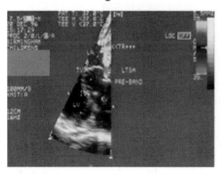
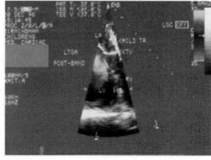

Figure 15.2 Echo images focusing on the position of the interventricular septum of a patient with ccTGA before and after PA banding. The shape of the septum changes from S-shaped to a straighter configuration, as emphasized by the solid lines below the images. (A black-and-white version of this figure will appear in some formats. For the colour version, please refer to the plate section.)

whom there is no prospect of ever converting to anatomical repair, are probably best treated with primary TV replacement; however, this is not always an easy decision because there is usually associated significant right ventricular dysfunction, and these can become high-risk procedures where even transplant might need to be considered. Operative risk depends on the underlying right ventricular function and associated lesions but is as high as 5 to 10 per cent in published series.

The Tricuspid Valve in Functionally Univentricular Circulations

Many functionally univentricular circulations will place the TV within the systemic position. The commonest situation is in hypoplastic left heart syndrome (HLHS; see Chapter 20), but it also occurs in unbalanced types of transposition/VSD or in double-outlet right ventricle (DORV) with a small LV. Again, the TV is most commonly structurally normal, but the globular shape of the RV and the septal attachments of the chordae predispose the TV to become regurgitant. The interaction between right ventricular dysfunction and TR can be difficult to unravel as the structure, shape and coronary supply of the RV are not as well adapted to cope at systemic pressures as the morphological LV. Nevertheless, some studies in HLHS have suggested that structural abnormalities of the TV do occur and may be as common as 20 to 30 per cent, especially in sub-types of HLHS with mitral atresia/aortic atresia. Timing of intervention and technique of repair will depend on the age of the patient and may be influenced by the timing of planned staged palliation of the underlying condition.

Surgical Management. Interventions on the TV in these patients are most commonly performed concomitantly with planned staged procedures in the univentricular pathway. Simple repair techniques as described earlier, such as annuloplasty and the Alfieri technique, are used most commonly, but in general, the results of repair are not as good as in the setting of a sub-pulmonary RV due to the inevitable increased strain, higher afterload and reduced compliance in the systemic RV. Concomitant progression from a volume-loaded circulation (such as Norwood or Blalock-Taussig (BT) shunt) to a cavo-pulmonary shunt or bidirectional Glenn shunt (Chapter 21) has the advantage of offloading the volume load on the systemic RV, which may improve the efficacy of repair

but will not abolish TR without also addressing the valve at the time of surgery. Repairs are still preferred in this group of patients since they are generally performed in children, with the need to allow for growth – but valve replacement with mechanical valves may be required in older patients or if the repair has failed. Again, the operative risk depends on the underlying right ventricular function – but most series report 5 to 10 per cent early mortality, reflecting the fact that many of these patients are in significant heart failure preoperatively.

Ebstein's Anomaly of the Tricuspid Valve

This complex anomaly of the TV is really an abnormality of the whole RV and valvar structure. The tricuspid valve is grossly abnormal such that the leaflets are corkscrewed or spiralled into the true ventricular cavity so that the TV no longer sits at the A-V junction. The traditional description of Ebstein's anomaly as being apical displacement of the septal leaflet of the TV is an oversimplification but does describe one of the characteristic features (Figure 15.3) of the lesion. The valve is spiralled into the ventricle to a variable degree, leaving part of the inferior and septal surfaces of the RV proximal to the valve and so functionally part of the atrium. These areas become very thin walled and are said to be 'atrialized' RV muscle. The leaflets themselves are very abnormal – with the septal leaflet displaced deeply down the septum, typically tethered and small and the inferior leaflet draped over the ventricular surface, usually covered in fenestrations and with very abnormal chordal

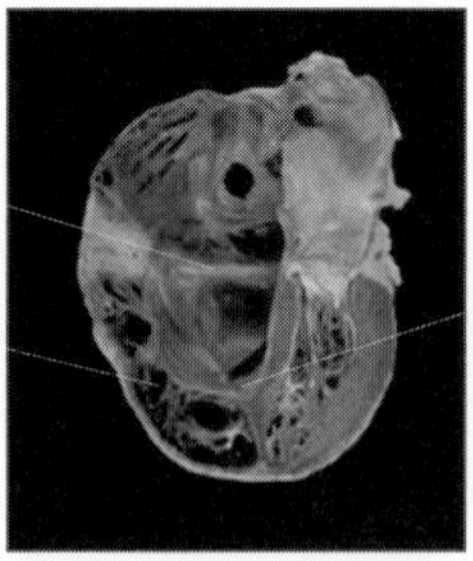

'Atrialized' Right Ventricle

Apical Displacement of the Tricuspid Valve

Figure 15.3 Ebstein's anomaly. The apical displacement of the tricuspid valve is clearly shown, creating a large 'atrialized' portion of the RV. The inferior leaflet of the TV is plastered along the free wall of the heart with multiple fibro-muscular connections, described as failed delamination of the valve.
Source: From Warnes CA et al. Journal of the American College of Cardiology : Volume 54, Issue 21, 17 November 2009, Pages 1903–1910. (A black-and-white version of this figure will appear in some formats. For the colour version, please refer to the plate section.)

attachments where the leaflet has failed to separate fully from the endocardium (so-called failed delamination) (Figure 15.3).

There is a great spectrum of Ebstein's anomaly, depending on the extent of the valvar displacement, with the most severe cases almost obliterating the functional cavity of the RV, many of these leading to

hydrops fetalis and early fetal loss. Severe cases that survive to birth can be profoundly unwell post-natally with a hugely enlarged heart shadow (the 'wall-to-wall heart'; Figure 15.4) occupying so much space that the lungs are small and underdeveloped, compounding the situation. These cases have severe TR with a very small right ventricular cavity and, if they survive, often have a functionally univentricular circulation (see below). Conversely, the remainder of the spectrum of Ebstein can remain remarkably symptom-free throughout childhood and tolerate the TR very well, some not presenting until adulthood. Associated ASD or accessory conduction pathways (leading to supra-ventricular tachycardias) may be the presenting feature.

Clinical Presentation and Investigation. Neonatal presentation should be considered separately since patients can be profoundly unwell and need immediate resuscitation. Severe cases are duct dependent and require prostaglandin E2 infusion and may need ventilatory support, often being severely cyanosed. Echocardiography will usually provide all the necessary information, particularly focusing on the size of the RV and on the flow across the pulmonary valve. CT scan may be helpful if there is concern over hypoplasia of the lungs in severe cases. The immediate management is to stabilize the situation and wait for 48 hours, if possible, as summarized in the flow

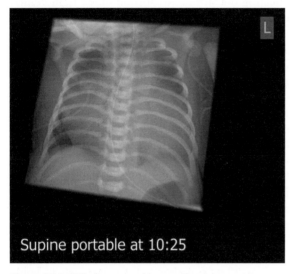

Supine portable at 10:25

Figure 15.4 CXR of neonate with sever Ebstein's anomaly showing a 'wall-to-wall heart'.

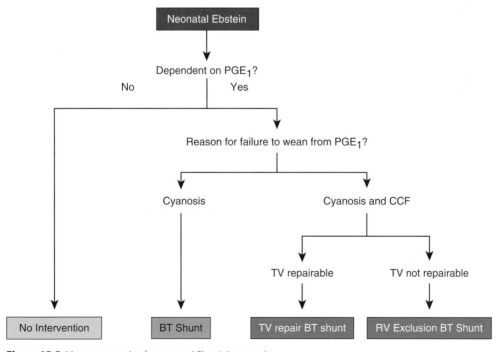

Figure 15.5 Management plan for neonatal Ebstein's anomaly.

diagram in Figure 15.5. As pulmonary vascular resistance (PVR) falls, the forward flow across the pulmonary valve may improve, and the physiology can improve dramatically. However, if patients remain duct dependent, then intervention will be required, as discussed below.

The majority of Ebstein's patients do not present as neonates and are usually remarkably well despite what can be severe regurgitation. Management is conservative, but patients need careful monitoring to track whether there is progression of TR, development of arrhythmias or deterioration in right ventricular function. The presence of an ASD can sometimes result in cyanosis if the regurgitant jet is directed through the defect and may become an indication for intervention. Although patients typically remain symptom free for many years, the natural history is not benign, and gradual deterioration in right ventricular function with progressive dilatation of the right atrium (RA – and RV) tends to occur. This progresses to variable degrees of dyskinesia of the interventricular septum and subsequent left ventricular dysfunction. Monitoring of both left and right ventricular function with echo and MRI is essential in older patients, and exercise testing can be a useful objective measurement of decline in function when considering referral for surgery. In the past, referral for surgical repair has often been delayed until patients were very symptomatic – but there is increasing evidence that referral should be made sooner, before there is deterioration in right ventricular function, particularly with the advent of better repair techniques.

Surgical Management. Neonatal management is summarized in Figure 15.5 and can be very high risk. Duct-dependent neonates may require a BT shunt with or without TV repair depending on the severity of regurgitation. Severe cases with no functional right ventricular cavity (i.e. severe Ebstein displacement of the valvar apparatus into the infundibulum of the RV, sometimes with associated pulmonary atresia) require BT shunt plus effective exclusion of the RV from the circulation; this is best achieved by patch closure of the tricuspid orifice, leaving a small hole in the patch to allow any coronary venous blood to escape and reducing the size of the giant RA (the 'Starnes procedure'). These procedures carry a 20 to 30 per cent mortality due to the preoperative state often being very fragile and due to the fact that the pulmonary arteries and lungs themselves can be small and poorly developed.

Management in older children and adults is elective and usually in the form of valve repair. Several types of repairs have been proposed that involved plicating the 'atrialized' portion of the right ventricular inferior wall and rotating or advancing the large anterior leaflet to coapt against the septum. The Carpentier and Danielson techniques were used most widely, with a 2 to 3 per cent operative mortality and a 60 to 70 per cent freedom from reintervention at 10 years. More recently, the 'cone repair' has gained widespread popularity with encouraging early results; the technique mobilizes the entire valve including the small septal leaflet and the tethered inferior leaflet to create a 360-degree 'cone' of leaflet tissue that is rotated back up to the true level of the A-V junction. The dilated tricuspid annulus is plicated, and the valve tissue is then reattached to the annulus at the anatomical level. This is the first technique that really restores the valve to the 'orthotopic' position, and early results show excellent function, but it is too early to know whether this will be sustained.

Overall outcomes of Ebstein repair are influenced mainly by the underlying right ventricular function. When ejection fraction (EF) falls to below 45 per cent, there is a significant deterioration in both early and late outcome. In patients with a severely dilated and poorly functioning RV, a concomitant cavopulmonary shunt has been performed in some patients. Patients late in the natural history who have developed secondary left ventricular dysfunction are also at increased operative risk. Older patients and those with severe right ventricular dysfunction may be better managed with primary TV replacement to avoid long cross-clamp times and complex repairs. Older patients also commonly have atrial fibrillation or flutter and require a concomitant Maze procedure, although restoration of sinus rhythm becomes less likely with age greater than 30 years. Earlier referral for surgery may avoid these higher-risk situations.

Transposition of the Great Arteries

William J. Brawn

Introduction

Transposition of the great arteries (TGA) accounts for about 10 per cent of children with congenital heart disease. The male-to-female ratio is 2:1. In TGA, the aorta arises from the morphological right ventricle (mRV), and the pulmonary artery (PA) arises from the morphological left ventricle (mLV). This is referred to as 'ventriculo-arterial (or V-A) discordance'. This means that the systemic venous return of desaturated blood passes from the right atrium (RA) through the tricuspid valve to the right ventricle (RV) and aorta. The oxygenated pulmonary venous return flows into the left atrium (LA) through the mitral valve into the left ventricle (LV) and PAs. Unless there is mixing of the blood at atrial, ventricular or ductal levels, the patient is inadequately oxygenated and dies. Most untreated patients die within the first few hours or days of life.

The external morphology of the heart is such that the aorta is positioned anterior and to the right of the PA, the so-called dextro-transposition or normal transposition (Figure 16.1). Associated cardiac malformations include ventricular septal defects (VSDs – peri-membranous or muscular), aortic arch coarctation/interruption and pulmonary stenosis. Overall, 60 to 70 per cent of all cases of TGA have an intact ventricular septum, 20 to 25 per cent have a VSD and the remaining 10 to 15 per cent are referred to as 'complex', implying a combination of VSD with arch anomalies or outflow tract stenosis.

Historically, patients survived only if there was as adequate-sized atrial or ventricular septal defect that allowed oxygenated and deoxygenated blood to mix. Surgical atrial septectomy, by Blalock and Hanlon (1950), followed by successful balloon atrial septostomy by Rashkind and Miller (1966) revolutionized the management of these patients, allowing mixing at the atrial level. Senning in 1959 and then Mustard in 1964 introduced an atrial baffling technique that re-directed the pulmonary venous return to the mRV and the systemic venous return to the mLV, thus restoring the normal physiological circulation. However, in this atrial switch, the mLV remained in the pulmonary circulation and the mRV in the systemic circulation. For the majority of patients, the mRV coped very well with the systemic circulation at first. However, the natural history for these patients has been the variable development of mRV failure and associated tricuspid regurgitation leading to congestive heart failure later in life.

True anatomic repair – i.e. restoring the mLV to the systemic circulation – was the goal, and in 1975, Jatene and colleagues described the first successful arterial switch procedure where the aorta and pulmonary artery were relocated to their respective left and right ventricles. The coronary arteries were also relocated to the new aorta in the same procedure. This

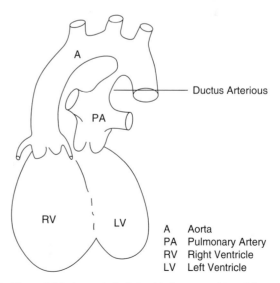

Figure 16.1 Anatomical relationship for transposition of the great arteries in dextro-TGA. The aorta is anterior and to the right, arising from the morphological right ventricle.

successful report set in train a change to the so-called arterial switch procedure for normal transposition. This also opened the possibility of infant repair, and in 1984, Castaneda in Boston and other centres reported successful neonatal repairs of TGA by the arterial switch procedure. The great advantage of the neonatal switch was that the LV could be restored to the systemic circulation before the ventricular muscle involuted and became weaker under the low-resistance pulmonary circuit. The other challenge in the arterial switch procedure is relocation of the coronary arteries. Unusual coronary artery patterns presented a technical challenge at the outset of the arterial switch procedure, but now different types of coronary artery patterns can be relocated in the arterial switch procedure without an increased risk.

Presentation and Diagnosis

Clinical presentation is usually of a very cyanosed sick baby, which occasionally may collapse and require urgent resuscitation. The standard form of resuscitation includes administration of prostaglandin E1 intravenously to reopen the duct and allow mixing at arterial level, correction of acid-base abnormalities and a balloon atrial septostomy often under echo Doppler control. Invariably, the baby can be stabilized with satisfactory systemic oxygen saturations after the balloon atrial septostomy. The prostaglandin E1 infusion may be stopped. Rarely, mixing is not adequate, and an emergency arterial switch is necessary. TGAs with and without VSDs are corrected by arterial switch within the first two weeks of life.

If there is no VSD, then the mLV will rapidly lose its muscle mass as it is working in the pulmonary circulation. Thus, it is essential that the arterial switch is performed before the mLV has begun to 'involute' in this way, necessitating surgery within the first two weeks of life. In rare cases of late presentation, the switch can be done at up to six to seven weeks of age, but the older the baby, the greater is the risk that the mLV will not cope in the systemic circulation (cases may need extra-corporeal membrane oxygenation (ECMO) support postoperatively or require 're-training' with the placement of a band on the PA). However, if there is a VSD, then the pressure in the mLV will be sustained, and it may be possible to delay the surgery for a few weeks – although in practice most centres would plan for repair within the first two weeks of life regardless. Other forms of TGA with arch and coarctation or interruption are also managed usually with a one-stage repair in the first two weeks of life. Where there is left ventricular outflow tract (LVOT) obstruction and VSD, the circulation may be well balanced and not need any initial intervention; however, if there is severe outflow tract obstruction, the pulmonary circulation is usually improved with a systemic shunt. Corrective surgery can usually be deferred until the first year or two of life.

Diagnosis is by echocardiography and (apart from the need in the majority for a balloon atrial septostomy to create a shunt at the atrial level) invasive investigation are not necessary. Echo Doppler can clearly define the great vessel anatomy, the presence of single or multiple VSDs, the presence of LVOT obstruction and aortic arch anomalies. In the presence of aortic arch anomalies, there may also be the potential for a RVOT obstruction beneath the aortic valve. In the great majority of cases, the coronary artery anatomy can be clearly defined as well. Occasionally, there are associated non-cardiac abnormalities that need addressing as well. The majority of cases are diagnosed post-natally, but antenatal diagnosis is increasing and can help in planning immediate management post-partum.

Arterial Switch Operation

The standard arterial switch procedure is performed through a midline sternotomy with atrial or bicaval venous cannulation with arterial return to the ascending aorta (or Gore-Tex tube for selective cerebral perfusion into the innominate artery in cases of associated arch problems). The heart is cardiopleged, and the fleshy, delicate ductus arteriosus is ligated, over-sewn and divided. The PAs are extensively dissected and looped with Silastic snares at the same time as the ductus arteriosus is delineated. The aorta is transected, and stay sutures are placed on the aortotomy adjacent to the commissures of the aortic valve. First the right coronary artery and then the left coronary artery are removed with cuffs of aortic wall tissue from the aortic root and relocated to incisions made in the old pulmonary artery. Different methods are used for this relocation, but medially hinged trapdoor incisions in the pulmonary artery are a reliable technique (Figure 16.2). Native pericardial patches are then sutured into the defects created by removal of the coronary arteries in the old aorta. At this point the PA bifurcation is mobilized anterior to the aorta (the 'Lecompte manoeuvre'), and the distal aorta is anastomosed to the new aorta as it leaves the heart from the mLV. The distal PA is then anastomosed to the old aorta and the new PA, anterior to the new ascending aorta (Figure 16.3). Relocation of the coronary arteries, in particular, coronary arteries that are of an abnormal or intra-mural cause, may be technically challenging and require readjustment to ensure unobstructed myocardial perfusion.

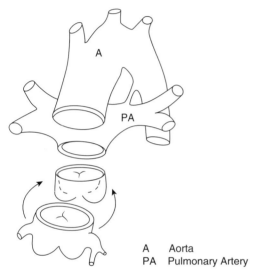

Figure 16.2 The arterial switch procedure. The great arteries have been transected above the level of the sino-tubular junction.

A   Aorta
PA   Pulmonary Artery

If a VSD is present, it is usually closed via the RA through the tricuspid valve. Unusually positioned VSDs may be closed via the old pulmonary root before the aorta is reconstructed or via a separate right ventriculotomy. Aortic arch reconstruction for coarctation or interruption is performed at the same time as the arterial switch to achieve an unobstructed aorta. It may be necessary to supplement the aortic reconstruction with a patch. Where there is coarctation or interruption of the aortic arch, there may be a small ascending aorta and aortic valve in association with some sub-aortic muscular stenosis, and this may require attention.

TGA with LVOT Obstruction

In TGA with LVOT obstruction, corrective surgery is usually deferred until the patient is older, usually in the second year of life, by increasing systemic oxygenation with a balloon septostomy and a systemic shunt (if necessary) in the neonatal period. Corrective surgery in this group of patients comprising re-routing of the VSD with a tunnel patch to the aorta and creating a PA-to-right-ventriculotomy connection with either a valve or a tube, the so-called Rastelli procedure (Figure 16.4). The PA can be relocated anterior to the aorta, as in the Lecompte manoeuvre, for classic normal transposition, and then a direct anastomosis is made between the PA and the right ventriculotomy usually with an anterior

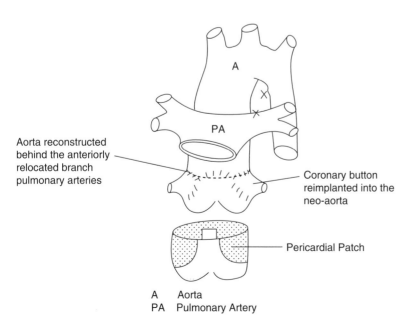

Figure 16.3 The coronary arteries have been excised from the original aorta and relocated into incisions made in the pulmonary root. The defects left in the original aorta are repaired with autologous pericardium.

Aorta reconstructed behind the anteriorly relocated branch pulmonary arteries

Coronary button reimplanted into the neo-aorta

Pericardial Patch

A   Aorta
PA   Pulmonary Artery

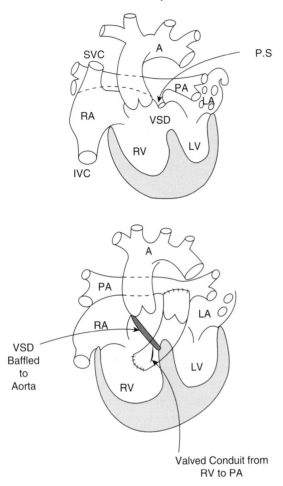

Rastelli Procedure for Transposition with Pulmonary Stenosis

Figure 16.4 The Rastelli procedure for correction of TGA with VSD and pulmonary stenosis/atresia.

patch of pericardium or valved conduit to restore continuity.

When the VSD is restrictive or in a difficult position to realign with the aorta with a patch, the Nikaidoh procedure can be performed (Figure 16.5). In this procedure, the aortic root and the coronary arteries are excised from the heart. The VSD is enlarged, and the aortic root is moved posteriorly into the pulmonary stenotic area, thus realigning the aorta in a straighter fashion to the left ventricular outflow tract. Pulmonary arteries are then reconnected to the right ventriculotomy with the Lecompte manoeuvre with or without patch supplementation.

Outcomes

The results of the arterial switch in the current era are extremely good with mortality approaching zero to 1 per cent for routine arterial switch with or without VSD closure. Associated arch anomalies increase the operative risk with a 5–10 per cent mortality in this 'complex' group. The most important risk factor is the presence of intra-mural coronary arteries which are only seen in 2–3 per cent of transpositions. TGA with VSD and pulmonary stenosis repairs via either the Rastelli, REV or Nikaidoh procedure also now have extremely good outcomes, with an operative risk of less than 5 per cent.

Long-Term Outcomes and Considerations

Restoration of the mLV to the systemic circulation in the arterial switch operation has revolutionized the management of patients with TGA. So far as can be seen, 20 to 30 years postoperatively, the results continue to be excellent, with well-functioning left and right ventricles. Early in most series there was a low incidence of problems with RVOT obstruction and PA stenosis, but this is no longer a major problem. The aortic valve, the old pulmonary valve, seems to be free of major problems, but there is a low incidence of increasing aortic valve regurgitation over time that occasionally requires aortic valve replacement (2 to 3 per cent of patients at 20 years). Likewise, in some patients, the proximal part of the aorta, the old pulmonary artery, dilates and may require root replacement.

Adult patients who in the past have undergone a Senning or Mustard procedure may have had problems with systemic or pulmonary venous pathway obstruction and mRV failure with tricuspid regurgitation. In young patients with these problems, there was a vogue for re-training the mLV with a PA band and then proceeding to an arterial switch. Whilst this was successful in some instances, the number of patients requiring this two-stage arterial switch is very small, and there are very few, if any, patients who now require this intervention.

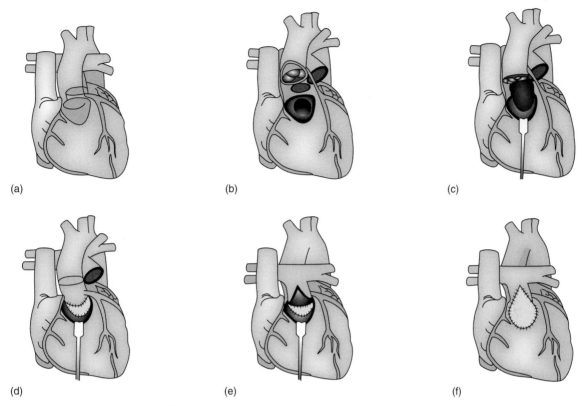

(a)   (b)   (c)

(d)   (e)   (f)

Figure 16.5 The Nikaidoh Procedure for repair of transposition with VSD and pulmonary stenosis/atresia (Artist please adapt). *Source*: Cardio Young 18: 124–34, 2008

Further Reading

Castaneda AR, Norwood WJ, Jonas RA et al. Transposition of the great arteries and intact ventricular septum; anatomical repair in the neonate. *Ann Thorac Surg* 1984; **38**: 438–43.

Co-Vn JG, Ginde S, Bartz PJ et al. Long term outcomes of the neoaorta after arterial switch operation for transposition of the great arteries. *Ann Thorac Surg* 2013; **95**(5): 1654–59.

Jaten AD, Fontes VF, Paulista PP et al. Successful anatomic correction of transposition of the great vessels: a preliminary report. *Arq Bras Cardiol* 1975; **28**: 461–64.

Fricke TA, d'Udekem Y, Richardson M et al. Outcomes of the arterial switch operation for transposition of the great arteries: 25 years of experience. *Ann Thorac* Surg 2012; **94** (1): 139–45.

Kalfa DM, Lambert V, Baruteau AE et al. Arterial switch for transposition with left outflow tract obstruction outcomes and risk analysis. *Ann Thorac Surg* 2013; **95**(6): 2097–103.

Lecompte Y, Zannini L, Hazan E et al. Anatomic correction of transposition of the great arteries. *J Thorac Cardiovasc Surg* 1981; **82**: 629–931.

Mee RBB. Severe right ventricular failure after Mustard or Senning operation: two-stage repair; pulmonary artery banding and switch. *J Thorac Cardiovasc Surg* 1986; **92**: 385–90.

Quaegebeur JM, Rotimer J, Brom AG et al. Revival of the senning operation in the treatment of transposition of the great arteries. *Thorac* 1977; **32**:517–24.

Trusler GA, Williams WG, Izukawa T et al. Current results with the Mustard operation in isolated transposition of the great arteries. *J Thorac Cardiovasc Surg* 1980; **80**: 381–89.

Double-Outlet Right Ventricle

David J. Barron

Introduction

This is one of the most complex morphological diagnoses in congenital heart disease as it requires clear 3D understanding of the intra-cardiac anatomy and consists of a spectrum of lesions that may require a variety of surgical solutions to achieve anatomical repair. The term 'double-outlet right ventricle' (DORV) means that there is a VSD and that both the great arteries are (predominantly) arising from the right ventricle. The aorta often overrides the VSD, but at least 50 per cent of the aorta must be committed to the RV in order to classify as a DORV. Usually, both ventricles are well developed, and complete biventricular repair depends on (1) the extent (if any) of any pulmonary or sub-pulmonary stenosis and (2) the relationship of the great vessels to the VSD. The essential components of the morphological spectrum of DORV are often best considered by appreciating the relationship of the aorta to the mitral valve – in the normal heart, these two structures are in direct fibrous continuity, but as the aorta moves anteriorly, it becomes more committed to the RV and further away from the mitral valve (Figure 17.1). Thus, the aorta sits on a complete skirt of muscle (an infundibulum). As the aorta moves further forward, it becomes even further away from the VSD than the pulmonary artery (PA) – continuing this anterior and rotational movement – and the great vessels become transposed in extreme cases of DORV.

Another way of classifying DORV is through the position of the VSD. The commonest orientation is the sub-aortic VSD, and the rarest is when the VSD is remote from both the great vessels – the non-committed VSD. Occasionally, the VSD is double committed, straddling beneath both the great vessels, and finally, as described earlier, the VSD can be sub-pulmonary, implying that the aorta is very anterior and distant from the LV.

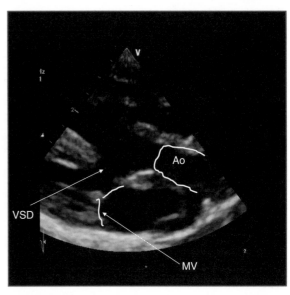

Figure 17.1 Long-axis parasternal view of DORV emphasizing the loss of continuity between the aortic (Ao) and mitral valve (MV).

Repair Options

Fallot with DORV. Part of the definition of tetralogy of Fallot is that the aorta overrides the ventricular septum; however, if the override is such that more than 50 per cent of the aorta is committed to the RV, then this is categorized as DORV. Often there is still direct continuity of the aorta to the MV, and the DORV is created in response to the deviation of the ventricular septum rather than the malposition of the aorta.

DORV with Unobstructed Right Ventricular Outflow Tract (RVOT). These patients will be in heart failure as for any patient with an unrestrictive VSD. Repair will depend on the relationship of the aorta to the VSD and requires an appreciation of the 3D pathway that will be created within the heart to commit the aorta back to the LV. In more severe cases, such a pathway may risk obstructing the outflow to the PA.

DORV with Sub-Pulmonary VSD. This implies a more severe form of DORV in that the aorta has moved so anteriorly that it is actually further away from the VSD than the PA (Figure 17.2). As a result, the great arteries are often malposed, being more side by side or even with the aorta anterior to the PA. This is known as the 'Taussig-Bing anomaly'. A decision has to be made as to whether the aorta can be baffled through to the VSD or an arterial switch would be preferable, then closing the VSD over to the (original) PA to achieve correction. The condition may also be associated with coarctation, aortic arch hypoplasia or aortic interruption (in around 50 per cent of cases).

DORV with Non-committed (Remote) VSD. This is rare, but occasionally the VSD is situated more in the inlet septum and is remote from the great vessels. The possibility of correction will depend on whether or not it is possible to create an adequate-sized pathway from the VSD to the aorta – thus correction depends on the size and exact position of the VSD. Some cases may not be septatable and need to consider a Fontan-type pathway.

Presentation and Diagnosis

Due to the spectrum of morphology, presentation essentially depends on the degree (or absence) of any pulmonary/sub-pulmonary stenosis. Patients with unobstructed pulmonary outflow will present similarly to a large VSD with congestive heart failure, breathlessness and failure to thrive. Those with moderate pulmonary stenosis may be well balanced (like an acyanotic Fallot), but more severe forms will be cyanosed to a varying degree. Patients who have associated coarctation of the aorta (CoA) or arch hypoplasia may present with circulatory collapse as the patent ductus arteriosus (PDA) closes in early neonatal life. Echocardiography will establish the diagnosis in all cases but may need careful and detailed study to elucidate the exact intra-cardiac anatomy. Careful assessment of the great vessel relationship and the position and size of the VSD is essential. The relationship of the aorta to the MV is also helpful. Echo alone is often sufficient, but in more complex cases, MRI and 3D reconstructions (even 3D printed models) can be helpful to understand whether or not the aorta is committable to the LV.

Management

Patients in heart failure can be stabilized with diuretics but usually need early surgical intervention. Complete repair in a single procedure is the preferred option but depends on the complexity of the intra-cardiac anatomy and any associated lesions.

Fallot with DORV. Management is as described in Chapter 11. Very cyanosed neonates may require palliation with a Blalock-Taussig (BT) shunt or RVOT

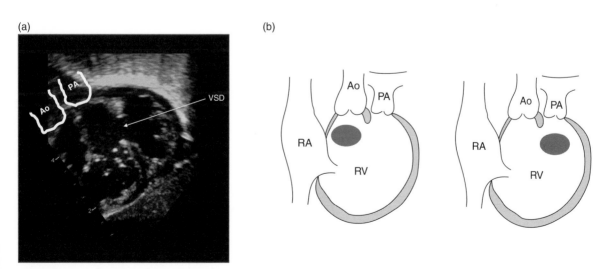

(a) (b)

Figure 17.2 (A) DORV with sub-pulmonary VSD showing the distance of the VSD from the aorta (aortic root = Ao; pulmonary root = PA). (B) Diagram showing the variable position of the VSD in the spectrum of DORV, showing a more sub-aortic position and a more sub-pulmonary position.

stent. Older infants are usually suitable to complete repair, Repair is essentially the same as for any Fallot, repairing the VSD in such a way as to commit the aorta back to the LV. Occasionally, it is necessary to enlarge the VSD to ensure that the pathway through to the aorta is not narrowed.

DORV with Unobstructed VSD. Simpler cases can be repaired as for any VSD, aiming for trans-atrial repair. However, if the aorta is very anterior, it may be necessary to perform a small right ventriculotomy to provide access to the upper margin of the VSD. In cases with greater displacement of the aorta the LV-aorta baffle may impinge on the outflow through to the PA, requiring additional enlargement of the sub-pulmonary area, usually with patch enlargement of the free wall of the infundibulum. Often, performing a small right ventriculotomy will both provide good access to the VSD and, by closing the ventriculotomy with a patch, will provide adequate size to the pulmonary outflow (Figure 17.3).

DORV with Sub-pulmonary VSD. This requires careful assessment. Most are usually best managed with arterial switch and then closing the VSD to the original PA, which is now the neo-aorta (Figure 17.4). The arterial switch can be difficult because of the side-by-side nature of the great vessels and the fact that unusual coronary artery patterns are found in 40 to 50 per cent of cases, but a Lecompte manoeuvre is usually possible. Associated arch hypoplasia further complicates the repair and can be addressed either as a single combined procedure or can be performed as a two-stage approach with initial arch repair and PA band. Single-stage repair is favoured, but outcomes with either strategy are similar. Older patients (usually after initial palliation with PA banding) can be considered for an intra-cardiac repair, baffling the VSD across to the aorta – known as the 'Kawashima operation' (Figure 17.5) – but need careful assessment to ensure that this is achievable without creating a long sub-aortic tunnel at the risk of subsequent stenosis.

DORV with Remote VSD. When the VSD is limited to the inlet and considerable distance from the aorta, it may not be possible to achieve repair. 3D assessments of the anatomy are helpful to establish whether it is possible to enlarge the VSD and baffle to the aorta.

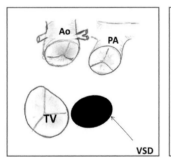
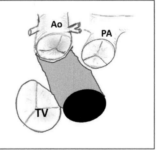

Figure 17.3 Diagram showing the relationship of the VSD to the valves within the heart as viewed from the RV in a case of DORV where the VSD can be tunnelled through to the aortic valve without obstructing the outflow through to the PAs.

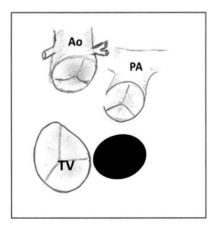
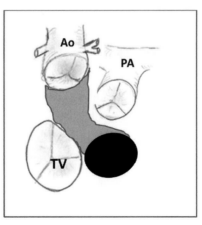

Figure 17.4 More severe case of DORV where the aorta has moved more anteriorly. The potential pathway of the VSD (shaded path) now risks narrowing the sub-aortic pathway.

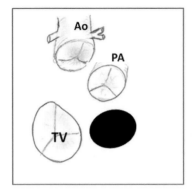 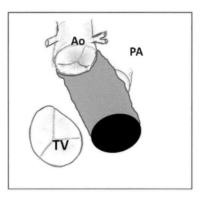 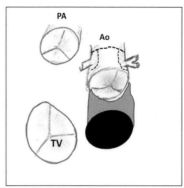

Figure 17.5 DORV with sub-pulmonary VSD. The aorta is now, anterior and an attempt to commit the VSD to the aorta (as shown in the middle panel with the shaded area) would risk obstructing the right outflow tract. An arterial switch, as shown in the final panel, allows the VSD to be committed with a more straightforward pathway.

Initial PA banding with a subsequent Fontan pathway may be the safest option.

Outcomes. Risks are higher than for simple VSD closure. Fallot with DORV carries a higher risk than 'simple' Fallot repair, with an operative risk of 4 to 5 per cent. Taussig-Bing outcome depends on associated arch pathology and the coronary patterns and carries an operative risk of 5 to 15 per cent. The need to enlarge the VSD leads to a risk of heart block of 5 to 10 per cent.

Associated arch obstruction can lead to difficult decision making as to a one- or two-stage repair. Despite a clear trend towards single-stage repair over the last 20 years, the outcomes with both strategies are similar. If a two-stage approach is chosen, then it is essential that the sub-aortic region is widely open because mal-alignment of the outlet septum can leave a substrate for sub-aortic obstruction.

Careful long-term follow-up is essential because the sub-aortic tunnel created by committing the aorta to the LV can lead to degrees of sub-aortic obstruction, with a need for late reoperation in 10 to 20 per cent.

Further Reading

Belli E, Serraf A, Lacour-Gayet F et al. Double-outlet right ventricle with non-committed ventricular septal defect. *Eur J Cardiothorac Surg* 1999; **15**(6): 747–52.

Bradley TJ, Karamlou T, Kulik A et al. Determinants of repair type, reintervention, and mortality in 393 children with double-outlet right ventricle. *J Thorac Cardiovasc Surg* 2007; **134**: 967–73.

Hayes DA, Jones S, Quaegebeur JM et al. Primary arterial switch operation as a strategy for total correction of Taussig-Bing anomaly: a 21-year experience. *Circulation* 2013; **10**(128)(11 Suppl 1): S194–98.

Kawashima Y, Fujita T, Miyamoto T, Manabe H. Intraventricular rerouting of blood for the correction of Taussig-Bing malformation. *J Thorac Cardiovasc Surg* 1971; **62**: 825–29.

Li S, Ma K, Hu S et al. Surgical outcomes of 380 patients with double outlet right ventricle who underwent biventricular repair *J Thorac Cardiovasc Surg* 2014; **148**(3): 817–24.

Soszyn N, Fricke TA, Wheaton GR et al. Outcomes of the arterial switch operation in patients with Taussig-Bing anomaly. *Ann Thorac Surg* 2011; **92**(2): 673–79.

Chapter 18

Congenitally Corrected Transposition of the Great Arteries

David J. Barron

Introduction

This complex condition is a type of transposition of the great arteries (TGA) and accounts for 2 per cent of all congenital heart disease, but it attracts a disproportionate amount of attention due to the unusual physiology and variety of associated conditions. The condition is characterized by atrio-ventricular (A-V) and ventriculo-arterial (V-A) discordance such that the physiology is naturally corrected in that the systemic venous blood is directed to the lungs and the pulmonary venous blood to the systemic circulation (Figure 18.1). However, in achieving this, the systemic ventricle is the morpho-logical right ventricle (mRV) and the sub-pulmonary ventricle is a morphologic left ventricle (mLV). The corrected physiology means that the patients are acyanotic and should be symptom free, but the clinical correlates are related to the high frequency of associated anomalies and the natural history of the mRV in the systemic position.

The associated conditions are listed in Table 18.1, with VSD being commonest at 60 per cent, together with the frequent combination of VSD with pulmon-ary stenosis or atresia (30 per cent in the Western world, up to 70 per cent in the East). The condition is also prone to conduction defects, with complete heart block developing in 40 per cent and abnormal-ities of the tricuspid valve (which is in the systemic circulation) causing regurgitation. The fascination with the condition is related to the natural history of the mRV in the systemic position, which is both unpredictable and partly dependent on the associated lesions.

Presentation

Presentation depends entirely on the associated lesions. Patients with a large VSD may present in heart failure, those with pulmonary stenosis or atresia will be cyanosed and those with arch hypo-plasia or coarctation may present with circulatory

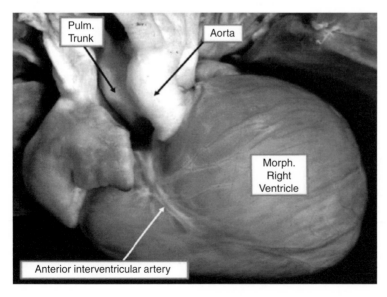

Pulm. Trunk

Aorta

Morph. Right Ventricle

Anterior interventricular artery

Figure 18.1 Heart with congenitally corrected transposition.
Source: Courtesy of Anderson R, *Cardiac Morphology.*
(A black-and-white version of this figure will appear in some formats. For the colour version, please refer to the plate section.)

Table 18.1 Associated Lesions in Congenitally Corrected Transposition of the Great Arteries (ccTGA) Undergoing Anatomical Repair[a]

Associated lesions/conditions	Frequency (%)
VSD	75–80
VSD and pulmonary stenosis/atresia	40–70[a]
Dextrocardia	20–25
Mesocardia	10–15
Situs inversus	5–7
DORV	5–7
Coarctation/arch hypoplasia	10–15
Ebsteinoid tricuspid valve	10–15
Bicuspid aortic valve	3
Abnormal mitral valve	3
Preoperative heart block	15–20

[a] There are considerable variations in the pattern of lesions seen based on geographical variation. The table reflects typical lesions seen in the western hemisphere. In the eastern hemisphere, LVOT obstruction with VSD is commoner with a lower incidence of arch hypoplasia and Ebsteinoid tricuspid valve.

collapse in the newborn period. Occasionally, patients are in complete heart block at birth and may present with heart failure secondary to profound bradycardia. Complete diagnosis can usually be made by echocardiography, and initial treatment is empirical, based on the nature of presentation to achieve a balanced circulation.

Patients with no significant associated lesions may be symptom free, and diagnosis may be made incidentally on a routine investigation such as an abnormal ECG (picking up conduction delay) or CXR (revealing an unusual position of the heart or the narrowed superior mediastinum characteristic of transposition). There are anecdotal cases diagnosed in their seventh or eighth decade, but most patients will develop some degree of right ventricular dysfunction (with or without tricuspid regurgitation) at some stage, with signs of congestive cardiac failure by age 50 in the majority of patients. Controversy remains over the management of symptom-less patients who develop echocardiographic signs of ventricular dysfunction and tricuspid regurgitation, and this is discussed later.

Initial Treatment

This will depend on the mode of presentation and the associated lesions: neonates with arch hypoplasia and coarctation require resuscitation, stabilization and urgent surgical repair. If there is associated VSD, then a pulmonary artery (PA) band may be placed at the same time to balance the circulation.

Patients with pulmonary stenosis or atresia require initial palliation with a Blalock-Taussig (BT) shunt, and those presenting with heart failure due to large VSD are usually initially managed with PA banding rather than VSD closure for reasons outlined below.

Conventional ('Physiological') Repair. Traditional management of ccTGA was to address the clinically important lesions and achieve a 'physiological' repair, closing any intra-cardiac shunts and relieving any outflow tract obstruction. This is referred to as a 'conventional repair' because it leaves the mRV as the systemic ventricle. Conditions such as ccTGA with pulmonary atresia and VSD are treated by simple VSD closure and placement of an LV-PA conduit (since the mLV is the sub-pulmonary ventricle). This approach is successful at relieving immediate symptoms, but the medium- to long-term outcomes are disappointing due to the tendency to develop right ventricular failure. The 10-year freedom from congestive heart failure after conventional repair is only 50 per cent, with a similar likelihood for greater than moderate tricuspid regurgitation. Attempts at tricuspid valve repair in this setting have been universally disappointing, with even experienced centres having a 100 per cent failure rate at 10 years. As a consequence, there is now far less enthusiasm for 'conventional' repair, but it is still appropriate in older patients, in whom the mRV function remains good.

Anatomical Repair. Concerns about the durability and function of the systemic right ventricle led to the concept of anatomical repair, restoring the mLV to the systemic position. This requires a more complex procedure that switches both the atrial pathways and the great arteries over, as well as addressing any associated lesions. Switching over the atrial pathways with an 'atrial switch' procedure is achieved with the Senning or Mustard procedure, which had been used in the 1960s to the early 1980s as a treatment for isolated TGA, only to be superseded by the arterial switch procedure.

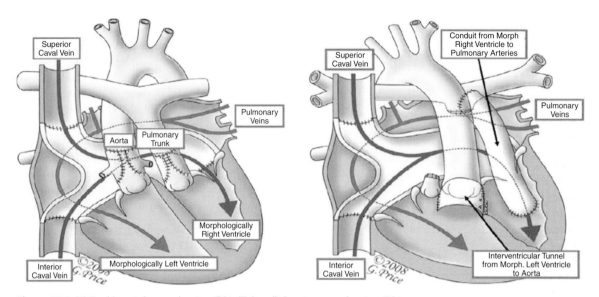

Figure 18.2 (A) Double-switch procedure in ccTGA. (B) Rastelli-Senning procedure in ccTGA.
Source: Courtesy of Anderson R, *Cardiac Morphology.*
(A black-and-white version of this figure will appear in some formats. For the colour version, please refer to the plate section.)

The great arteries are switched over with an arterial switch procedure or with a Rastelli procedure for patients with pulmonary stenosis or atresia (Figure 18.2). Thus, these anatomical repairs of ccTGA are generally referred to as 'double-switch procedures', sometimes further divided into the 'double-switch procedure' and the 'Rastelli-Senning procedure' according to the LVOT morphology. These are very complex procedures requiring long cross-clamp times, but they have been achieved with an operative mortality of 3 to 5 per cent. Outcomes have been encouraging, with the mLV having been restored to the systemic position generating much improved middle and late outcomes compared to conventional repair. The techniques have led to the renaissance of the atrial switch procedures, which would otherwise have become almost redundant. However, the techniques are not without problems, and the atrial switch technique can lead to baffle obstructions and atrial arrhythmias later in life. Also, the atrial switch component can lead to aortic regurgitation and branch pulmonary artery stenosis during follow-up; this is partly because the operations are generally performed at a much later age than the neonatal switch, and the potential for distortion of the great vessels is increased. It may not be possible to perform the Lecompte manoeuvre in this older age group, leaving the pulmonary arteries behind the aorta.

Late dysfunction of the mLV following anatomical repair has been reported and appears to be commoner in those corrected at a later age. Re-synchronization therapy may help in some cases.

Pulmonary Artery Banding and 'Re-Training'. Given the success of anatomical repair, there has been a move towards achieving anatomical repair wherever possible. For this to be possible, the mLV has to be capable of working against the systemic vascular resistance. In situation where the mLV has always been sustained at systemic pressures (such as in the presence of a large VSD or in pulmonary atresia), this is not a problem. However, there are situations in older children with no (or a small) VSD and no LVOT obstruction where the mLV has become used to working at lower pressures and has undergone a degree of involution. In these cases, anatomical repair is not possible because the mLV would fail when exposed to the systemic resistance. This led to the concept of banding the PA to create an iatrogenic afterload on the mLV and so elicit a pathophysiological response in both muscular hypertrophy and structure that would 're-train' the mLV and allow subsequent anatomical repair to become possible.

Thus, in the spectrum of ccTGA, PA banding is used for two indications:

1. To protect the pulmonary vasculature. In the setting of a large VSD, this is a more standard use

of a band to balance the Qp:Qs and prevent congestive cardiac failure. In this setting, the mLV will have always been maintained at systemic pressure (due to the large VSD) and does not require 're-training'.

2. To 're-train' the mLV. There is no VSD or only a small VSD, and the band is placed to stress the mLV and stimulate hypertrophy to prepare for subsequent anatomical repair. The response of the mLV to the band can be unpredictable, and it may not be possible to achieve this is a single procedure. Re-banding may be necessary to gradually increase afterload, although the advantage of banding in a growing child is that the band will naturally become 'tighter' as the child grows. The additional advantage of banding is that the higher pressure in the mLV leads to realignment of the interventricular septum, which, in turn, may stabilize the tricuspid valve and reduce tricuspid regurgitation. Thus, banding itself may be therapeutic in the sense that it can reduce tricuspid regurgitation.

The concept of PA banding to re-train remains controversial. Response to the band can be unpredictable, and the duration necessary to achieve re-training can also vary. Some cases are unable to achieve systemic pressure, and some need re-banding to achieve this; some never can. Assessment of readiness for anatomical repair is still poorly understood but can be aided by measurements of LV free-wall thickness and angiography with and without dobutamine stress. Most re-training is achieved within 18 months. There is concern that the older the patient is, the more difficult it is to re-train and that the long-term performance of the re-trained LV is not as good as the LV that has always been maintained at systemic pressure. It seems unlikely that re-training can be achieved beyond the age of 13 years, and most successful cases are banded in early childhood. Nevertheless, PA banding may have a 'third' role in splinting the interventricular septum, reducing or at least preventing progression of tricuspid regurgitation and so treating heart failure in patients with a failing mRV but too old to consider anatomical repair.

The Problem of Adult Uncorrected Cases. One of the many perplexing problems of ccTGA is that patients can remain entirely symptom free in early life but present later as the mRV starts to fail in combination with increasing tricuspid regurgitation – the relationship between the two events being closely interrelated. These patients are too old to consider re-training but may benefit from 'therapeutic' PA banding, as discussed earlier. Tricuspid valve repair in this setting is unlikely to be successful, but there has been some success for tricuspid valve replacement as long as right ventricular ejection fraction is still maintained (>45 per cent), but in general, adult patients who develop right ventricular failure may end up on a transplant programme. There is also a role for re-synchronization therapy in ccTGA patients who are pacemaker dependent due to associated heart block.

Further Reading

Barron DJ, Jones TJ, Brawn WJ. The Senning procedure as part of the double-switch operations for congenitally corrected transposition of the great arteries. *Semin Thorac Cardiovasc Surg Pediatr Card Surg Annu* 2011; **14**: 109–15.

Devaney EJ, Charpie JR, Ohye RG, Bove EL. Combined arterial switch and Senning operation for congenitally corrected transposition of the great arteries: patient selection and intermediate results. *J Thorac Cardiovasc Surg* 2003; **125**: 500–7.

Gaies MG, Goldberg CS, Ohye RG et al. Early and intermediate outcome after anatomic repair of congenitally corrected transposition of the great arteries. *Ann Thorac Surg* 2009; **88**: 1952–60.

Horer J, Schreiber C, Krane S et al. Outcome after surgical repair/palliation of congenitally corrected transposition of the great arteries. *Thorac Cardiovasc Surg* 2008; **56**: 391–97.

Hraska V, Mattes A, Haun C et al. Functional outcome of anatomic correction of corrected transposition of the great arteries. *Eur J Cardiothorac Surg* 2011; **40**(5): 1227–34.

Langley SM, Winlaw DS, Stumper O et al. Midterm results after restoration of the morphologically left ventricle to the systemic circulation in patients with congenitally corrected transposition of the great arteries. *J Thorac Cardiovasc Surg* 2003; **125**: 1229–41.

Malhotra SP, Reddy VM, Qiu M et al. The hemi-Mustard/bidirectional Glenn atrial switch procedure in the double-switch operation for congenitally corrected transposition of the great arteries: rationale and midterm results. *J Thorac Cardiovasc Surg* 2010; **141**(1): 162–70.

Murtuza B, Barron DJ, Stumper O et al. Anatomic repair for congenitally corrected transposition of the great arteries: a single-institution 19-year experience. *J Thorac Cardiovasc Surg* 2011; **142**(6): 1348–57.

Myers PO, del Nido PJ, Geva T et al. Impact of age and duration of banding on left ventricular preparation before anatomic repair for congenitally corrected transposition of the great arteries. *Ann Thorac Surg* 2013; **96**(2): 603–10.

Shin'oka T, Kurosawa H, Imai Y et al. Outcomes of definitive surgical repair for congenitally corrected transposition of the great arteries or double outlet right ventricle with discordant atrioventricular connections: risk analyses in 189 patients. *J Thorac Cardiovasc Surg* 2007; **133**: 1318–28.

Wilcox BR, Cook AC, Anderson RH. Surgical Anatomy of the Heart. Cambridge University Press, 2004.

Truncus Arteriosus

William J. Brawn

Introduction

Truncus arteriosis is a congenital heart condition where there is a single arterial outlet from the heart, the so-called truncus, which then divides into the aorta and the pulmonary artery (PA). The condition makes up 3 per cent of all congenital heart defects. It is thought that during development of the heart, there is failure of separation of the PA from the aorta, which are both derived from the primitive truncal vessel. The PA can arise as a single opening from the trunk and then divides into left and right PAs (type 1 truncus in the Van Praagh classification; Figure 19.1). The left and right PAs may arise as two separate vessels (type 2). Rarely, a ductus arteriosus supplies the left PA, and the right PA alone arises from the truncus vessels (type 3). In some 60 per cent of cases, the aorta is to the left side of the trachea, and 30 per cent are located to the right side. In about 10 per cent of cases there is an interruption of the aortic arch between the left carotid arteries and the left subclavian arteries (type 4). Coarctation of

the aorta is extremely rare. The coronary arteries usually arise in their usual positions from the sinuses of the truncal vessel above the truncal valve, but there can be a lot of variability in the origin of these vessels and their pathways to the myocardium. Truncus arteriosus is associated in the vast majority of patients with a large, unrestrictive sub-arterial ventricular septal defect (VSD). In the majority of cases, the truncal valve is tricuspid and neither stenotic nor incompetent. The truncal valve, however, shows great variability in morphology and can be bicuspid or quadri-cuspid and in these cases quite dysplastic. In particular, the quadri-cusp valve can be incompetent and stenotic. Management of the truncal valve in these situations is a surgical challenge. Rarely, the left ventricle in this condition is small, merging towards the hypoplastic left heart spectrum of conditions. These patients may require univentricular repair. As with other congenital heart conditions with aortic arch problems, DiGeorge syndrome is a common association. Therefore, irradiated blood products are recommended in managing these patients in an attempt to avoid graft-versus-host sensitization. In association with the DiGeorge syndrome, there may be problems with calcium metabolism, and calcium supplementation may be needed.

Diagnosis and Presentation

Diagnosis is invariably made by echocardiography alone without the need for invasive cardiac catheterization. If more information is needed to define the morphology of the aorta and PAs, then a CT scan or MRI may be advised. Often the diagnosis is made antenatally by maternal-fetal scans. The non-invasive investigations can define the underlying anatomy, the presence of the VSD, the single origin of the great vessel from the heart and the presence of aortic arch anomalies. The underlying ventricular function can also be assessed. It is important to define as clearly as possible the morphology and function of the truncal valve.

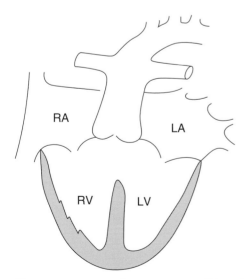

Figure 19.1 Anatomy of truncus arteriosus (RA = right atrium; LA = left atrium; RV = right ventricle; LV = left ventricle).

Clinically, these patients present with congestive cardiac failure. Whilst they may be quite stable for the first few days or week or two of life with high post-natal pulmonary vascular resistance (PVR), as the PVR falls, the left-to-right shunt through the VSD increases volume loading the heart and creating heart failure. Complicating this picture is the diastolic runoff to the low-resistance pulmonary vascular bed, so the diastolic pressure can be very low. This creates a steal of blood from the coronary arteries and can cause severe myocardial ischaemia with associated changes on ECG. These patients are susceptible to sudden cardiac arrest because of myocardial ischaemia, and even when resuscitated, this can be repeated. Clinically, then, these patients are in low cardiac output, congestive cardiac failure with high pulmonary blood flow because of the diastolic runoff to the pulmonary arteries and left-to-right shunt through the VSD. They are usually very tachypnoeic. They fail to thrive and do not gain weight. They are susceptible to sudden death. For this reason, these patients remain in hospital and are operated upon as soon as possible to correct the truncus arteriosus abnormalities.

Patients who are not diagnosed because they do not develop these symptoms may be diagnosed because of continuing high PVR, and they may go on to develop pulmonary vascular disease later in life and because of this become inoperable. This is a very rare situation in the developed countries.

Medical and Surgical Management

Having made the diagnosis, with the patient in hospital and whilst awaiting surgery, the baby can be managed with diuretics and angiotensin-converting enzyme (ACE) inhibitors. Supplemental oxygen may be required, and the children may be best managed on the intensive care unit with or without ventilation. However, these are only temporizing measures prior to urgent surgery.

Surgery comprises of (Figure 19.2)

1. Separation of the pulmonary arteries from the truncal vessel to create a separate aorta and pulmonary artery system.
2. Ventricular septal closure to the aorta.
3. Reconstruction of a connection between the right ventricular and pulmonary arteries, usually with a valved conduit, but an alternative is to bring the PAs directly onto the ventriculotomy and roof the outflow tract over with a patch (typically bovine pericardium).
4. Reconstruction of the aortic arch in the case of interruption of the aorta.
5. In patients with severe truncal valve abnormalities it may be necessary to repair the valve.

The details of the operation vary from patient to patient depending on morphology. Arterial cannulation is beneath the innominate artery in the truncal vessel with either bicaval or single venous cannulation of the right atrium. In my practice, the patient is usually cooled to 25°C nasopharyngeal. The majority of the operation is performed on cardiopulmonary bypass. In unusual circumstances with difficulty in accessing the VSD or the arch vessels, the patient may be cooled to below 18°C nasopharyngeal and then circulatory arrest used (direct cannulation via a Gore-Tex tube anastomosed to the innominate

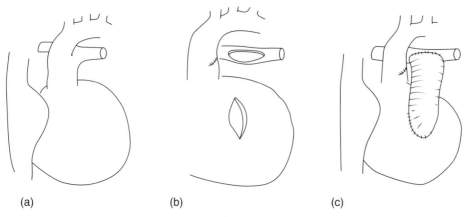

(a)   (b)   (c)

Figure 19.2 Repair of truncus arteriosus. (A) Initial anatomy with the pulmonary arteries arising from the leftward side of the trunk. (B) Pulmonary arteries disconnected from the trunk; the defect has been closed by direct suture. A vertical right ventriculotomy has been made to access the VSD, which is closed with a patch. (C) The RV has been connected to the pulmonary arteries using a homograft valved conduit.

artery to allow selective cerebral perfusion can be used if arch reconstruction is also required). The left and right PAs are occluded to prevent cardiopulmonary bypass runoff into the lungs, the truncal vessel is clamped, and the heart cardiopleged. The pulmonary arteries are excised from the back of the truncal vessel, and the defect in the trunk is directly sutured. Where there is a large defect in the trunk, this can be patched (usually with bovine pericardium) or, when there is separation of the left and pulmonary arteries to the lateral margins of the trunk, the truncal vessel itself may be completely transected, excising the left and right PAs on a ribbon of truncal wall posteriorly, and then the new aorta is reconstructed by direct anastomosis. A ventriculotomy is performed in the outflow tract of the right ventricle. The VSD is visualized and closed usually with a bovine pericardial patch held in position with interrupted 6-0 Prolene bovine pericardial pledgetted sutures, although a continuous suture is used successfully in many centres and different types of patch material can be used. This patch re-routes the VSD to the new aortic valve, the old truncal valve. The PAs are then connected to the RV, usually with a valve conduit, a donated homograft if available, either pulmonary or aortic, or a tissue valve such as a Contegra (Medtronic) valve (Figure 19.2C).

These patients are small, and the availability of small valves in this group makes it difficult always to acquire a valved conduit. Therefore, when the truncal valve, the new aortic valve, is functioning well, we will directly connect the PAs to the right ventriculotomy, patching over either with a mono-cusp valve or a direct bovine pericardial patch (Figure 19.3). If the truncal valve needs attention, this is addressed when the trunk is open. Usually the problem is one of truncal incompetence, and this can be improved by re-suspending the prolapsing small leaflets of the usually quadra-cuspid valve by direct anastomosis of these leaflets to a supporting cusp of a large cusp with a well-formed sinus that is well supported by its commissures. This usually creates a bicuspid valve that is sometimes mildly stenotic but less incompetent. This new aortic valve may function very well for many months or years but may require replacement with a mechanical valve in an older patient or an aortic root replacement with a donated homograft in some instances. Also, when the truncal root is open, the origins of the coronary arteries need to be identified and their pathways to the myocardium carefully probed to identify intramural coronary arteries or unusual pathways. In reconstructing the new aorta, care has to be taken not to distort the coronary arteries.

When truncus arteriosus is associated with aortic arch interruption, this is also repaired at the same time, usually with isolated cerebral perfusion by cardiopulmonary bypass. The reconstruction is usually supplemented by a patch of homograft material to allow an unobstructed pathway from the heart to the descending thoracic aorta.

Postoperative Management. Patients can be fragile postoperatively (particularly if unstable prior to surgery) and require careful monitoring of the left atrial pressure and judicious use of diuretics and inotropic support. Patients exposed to very high pulmonary

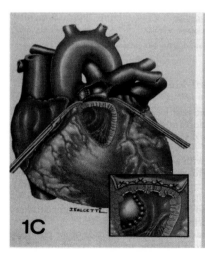

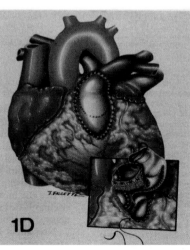

Figure 19.3 Direct anastomosis of the pulmonary arteries to the ventriculotomy. The defect is then roofed over with a patch, avoiding the need for a valved conduit. *Source:* From Barbero-Marcial et al. A technique for correction of truncus arteriosus types I and II without extracardiac conduits. *Journal Thoracic Cardiovascular Surgery* 1990; 99: 364–69. (A black-and-white version of this figure will appear in some formats. For the colour version, please refer to the plate section.)

blood flow preoperatively, and particularly for some time (i.e. older neonates), may be at risk of pulmonary hypertensive crises in the postoperative period. Direct measurement of PA pressures (with a monitoring line placed at the time of surgery) may be necessary in such patients to track changes in pressure and guide treatment. Pulmonary hypertensive crises are treated with ventilating with 100 per cent oxygen, decreasing the partial pressure of carbon dioxide (pCO_2), use of pulmonary vasodilators such as milrinone and the use of inhaled nitric oxide (iNO). All my patients having this procedure have the sternum left open for the first 24 to 48 hours after surgery, and then the chest is formally closed in the intensive care unit a day or two after the repair. The peri-operative mortality for this group of patients when there is no associated problems with the truncal valve or the aortic arch is 7 to 10 per cent, but with associated problems it rises to 15 per cent.

Follow-up

In general, these patients do very well, with one-year survival now approaching 90 per cent. Those with DiGeorge syndrome require closer surveillance and may have developmental delay. The main issue relates to the nature of the reconstruction of the connection of the RV to the PAs, and these patients do require reoperations to replace valved conduits or reconstruct the right ventricular outflow tract over the years ahead. Freedom from surgical replacement of the RV-PA conduit is 50 to 60 per cent at five years, but if no conduit is used, the reoperation rate is much less. Likewise, any problems with the truncal valve may also need addressing either with a root replacement or a mechanical aortic valve replacement.

Further Reading

Bove EL, Beekman RH, Snider AR et al. Repair of Truncus arteriosus in the neonate and young infant. *Ann Thorac Surg* 1989; **47**: 499–505.

Crupi G, Macartney FJ, Anderson RH. Persistant truncus arteriosus. A study of 66 autopsy cases with special reference to definition and morphogenesis. *Ann J Cardiol* 1977; **40**: 569–78.

McElhinney DB, Reddy VM, Rajasinghe HA et al. Trends in the management of truncal valve insufficiency. *Ann Thorac Surg* 1998; **65**: 517–24.

Russell HM, Pasquadi SK, Jacocbs JP et al. Outcomes of repair of common arterial trunk with truncal valve surgery: a review of the Society of Thoracic Surgeons Congenital Heart Surgery Database. *Ann Thorac Surg* 2012; **93**(1): 164–69.

Chapter 20

Hypoplastic Left Heart Syndrome

William J. Brawn

Introduction

The term 'hypoplastic left heart syndrome' was coined by Noonan and Nadas in 1958 to describe a very characteristic underdevelopment of the left side of the heart. Classically, it comprises a very small or diminutive ascending aorta in association with severe aortic stenosis or aortic atresia and mitral stenosis or atresia. There is variable underdevelopment of the left ventricle and usually associated hypoplasia of the aortic arch with coarctation of the aorta. Physiologically, the systemic circulation is supported by the right ventricle (RV) with blood flow through a patent ductus arteriosus (PDA) supplying the systemic circulation. The majority of patients die within a few hours or days of birth when the ductus arteriosus closes and the systemic circulation is stopped (Figure 20.1). Whilst hypoplastic left heart syndrome is rare, a 2 to 3 per cent of all congenital defects, untreated it is responsible for about 30 per cent of neonatal cardiac deaths. No definite cause for the condition has been found, although in a minority of cases some chromosomal abnormalities are associated with this condition (e.g. Jacobsen syndrome)

Whilst hypoplastic left heart syndrome represents the more severe end of the spectrum of hypoplasia of the left heart, there can be a variable degree of hypoplasia of the left ventricle, left ventricular outflow tract and mitral valve in association with aortic arch anomalies. Much of the decision making as to possible surgery for this condition relates to deciding whether or not the left side is big enough to support the systemic circulation; in other words, can the heart be septated into left and right ventricles?

Pathophysiology

The management of hypoplastic left heart syndrome was revolutionized in the 1970s and 1980s by the introduction of prostaglandin into paediatric cardiology practice in order to maintain patency of the ductus arteriosus. At the same time, intensive care management of very sick neonates improved dramatically, and it was possible to keep these children alive for possible surgical interventions. The hypoplasia of the left ventricle and aorta means that the systemic circulation cannot be supported in the usual way by the left heart, and the systemic perfusion depends on blood flow through a PDA. This duct can be kept open with prostaglandin and the child either resuscitated or, if diagnosed antenatally, prevented from collapse.

In the 1980s, Bill Norwood in Boston Children's Hospital pursued a surgical programme to attempt to palliate these babies and developed the three-stage

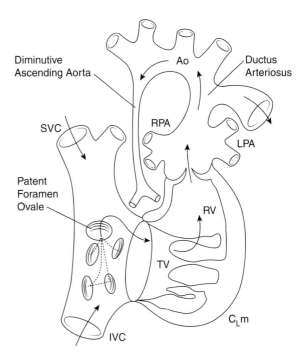

Figure 20.1 Diagram of hypoplastic left heart syndrome (Ao = aorta; SVC = superior vena cava; IVC = inferior vena cava; TV = tricuspid valve; RV = right ventricle; PVs = pulmonary veins; LPA = left pulmonary artery; RPA = right pulmonary artery).

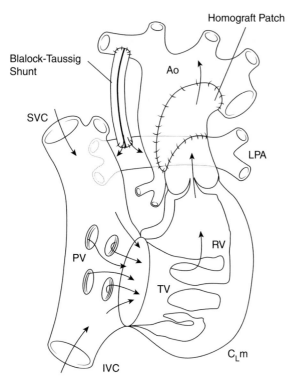

Figure 20.2 Diagram of 'classical' Norwood I procedure with modified BT shunt.

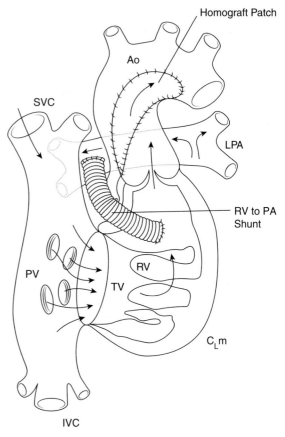

Figure 20.3 Diagram of Norwood I procedure with RV-to-PA conduit.

Norwood procedure. This procedure and its derivatives are used by most congenital heart centres now. Other methods of treatment such as the hybrid procedure and cardiac transplantation are also used but only in a small number of centres.

Norwood Procedure

Classically, the Norwood procedure has three components. The first stage, performed in the first few days of life, comprises a reconstruction of the systemic outflow tract from the heart by connecting the pulmonary artery to the aorta. Blood flow to the lungs is achieved by a modified Blalock-Taussig (BT) shunt in the classical Norwood procedure (Figure 20.2); more recently, many centres are using a direct RV-to-PA conduit (Figure 20.3). At the same procedure, an open atrial septectomy is performed so that there is no restriction of blood flow from the pulmonary veins into the RV. The circulation thus comprises systemic and pulmonary venous return, mixing in a common atrial chamber, and passing through the tricuspid valve into the right ventricular outflow tract and then to the systemic circulation. This systemic circulation also supplies the pulmonary blood flow, either by the BT shunt or by the RV-to-PA conduit.

The Norwood II procedure is performed at about four to six months of age. At that time, the BT shunt or RV-to-PA conduit is removed, and the pulmonary circulation is restored by connecting the SVC to the PA, either by a direct SVC-to-PA anastomosis (Figure 20.4) or by partial septation of the upper part of the atrial chamber to create the so-called hemi-Fontan procedure (Figure 20.5).

The final stage, Norwood II or the Fontan procedure, is performed in our unit at about four to six years of age; in some other units, it is done when patients are younger. It comprises the connection of the IVC directly to the PAs, usually with an external prosthetic tube of about 20 mm in diameter (Figure 20.6). Thus, all the systemic venous return flows into the pulmonary circulation. There is separation from the oxygenated from the deoxygenated blood, and the patient is almost fully saturated.

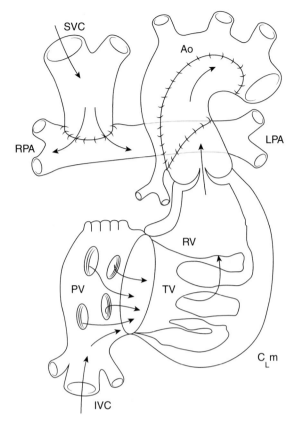

Figure 20.4 Diagram of bidirectional cavo-pulmonary shunt in the Norwood II procedure.

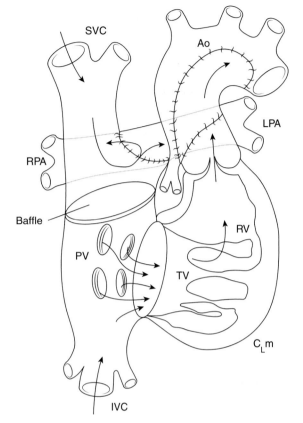

Figure 20.5 Diagram of hemi-Fontan procedure for Norwood II.

Outcome

As one might imagine with this complex surgery, there is mortality, but it largely revolves around the stage I procedure performed in the first few days of life, with a mortality of about 15 per cent. The mortality for the stages II and III approaches zero in the current era. Complications related to the procedures are recurrence of coarctation of the aorta and poor right ventricular function, often associated with varying degrees of tricuspid regurgitation, restrictive pulmonary flow through the BT or RV-to-PA shunts and development of sepsis related to the shunt in particular, with an association of low cardiac output and shunt occlusion. In general, in the stage II Norwood, the cavo-pulmonary shunt, and stage III, the Fontan procedure, are pretty much free of problems excepting for fluid collection on the lungs after the Fontan procedure, which may be troublesome for two to three weeks after the surgery. In an attempt to diminish this problem, many centres leave a small communication ('fenestration') between the atrium and the external conduit to prevent high pressures in the pulmonary circulation after the Fontan procedure.

Hybrid Procedure and Cardiac Transplantation

Because of the initial high mortality and the morbidity associated with the Norwood procedure and the difficulty in managing babies presenting in severe low cardiac output, other methods were developed to overcome these problems. The main one is that of the so-called hybrid procedure, where the major surgery is avoided in the first few weeks of life by maintaining duct patency either with chronic administration of prostaglandin or with placement of a stent into the duct together with placement of bilateral left and right PA bands to restrict pulmonary flow and balance the systemic pulmonary circulation. This method has been applied in our

93

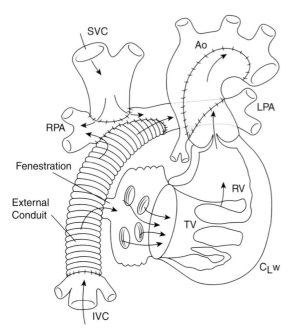

Figure 20.6 Diagram of total cavo-pulmonary connection (TCPC) or Fontan completion using external conduit from IVC to PAs with fenestration.

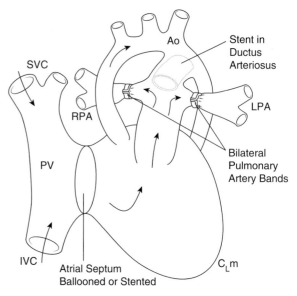

Figure 20.7 Diagram of neonatal palliation using hybrid technique.

own unit when a child presents in a very bad state and would not be suitable for a Norwood I procedure without resuscitation by the hybrid procedure. Other centres have used this method as a primary procedure, followed by the so-called combined stage II, where the arch is repaired, the stents removed, the bands removed and a direct cavo-pulmonary anastomosis is performed as for the Norwood II. The child then progresses through to the Fontan procedure in the usual way.

Heart transplantation for these patients was popularized in the early period by a group at Loma Linda, where neonatal hearts were available. However, in general terms, donors are not available in sufficient numbers to provide a suitable source for this group of patients.

Peri-operative Progress

The management of the peri-operative period in stage I Norwood patients can be particularly difficult and has extended the efforts of neonatal intensive care greatly. It is worth noting that we have learnt much in the way from managing patients with hypoplastic left heart syndrome (HLHS) that we can use in other neonates with severe cardiac problems.

The majority of deaths with HLHS occur in the first few weeks of life after the Norwood I procedure. Stages II and III have a very low operative mortality and morbidity, and survival at one year now approaches 75 per cent. Thereafter, in the early years, there is very little mortality or morbidity related to this syndrome managed in this way.

Comment

There is little doubt that the surgery for HLHS and its variants has had an impact not only on the outcome to these children but also on other neonates with similar difficult problems by virtue of the overall management of children with a hypoplastic left heart. The mortality over the last 20 years has fallen quite dramatically, and the actuarial survival at one year approaches 75 per cent. Early on in the development of this programme, there was a large amount of morbidity related to the immediate peri-operative management of patients with cerebral morbidity as well as local cardiac morbidity related to the surgery. However, over the years, this has gradually fallen, with improved results for the Norwood I procedure. The Fontan procedure has its own complications related to the high pressure (14 mmHg) in the pulmonary and systemic venous circulations together with lack of pulmonary pulsatile flow. These can include congested liver leading to cirrhosis, protein-losing enteropathy, pulmonary embolization, heart failure and cardiac arrhythmias. As a result, the long-term outcome over 20 to 40 years of this complex surgical programme is as yet unknown.

Further Reading

Barron DJ, Kilby MD, Davies B et al. Hypoplastic left heart syndrome. *Lancet* 2009; **374**(9689): 551–64.

McGuirk SP, Griselli M, Stumper O et al. Staged surgical management of hypoplastic left heart syndrome in a single institution 12 year experience. *Heart* 2006; **92**: 364–70.

Norwood WI, Lang P, Hansen DD. Physiologic repair of aortic atresia: hypoplastic left heart syndrome. *N Engl J Med* 1983; **308**: 23–26.

Sano S, Ishino K, Kawada M et al. Right ventricle–pulmonary artery shunt in first stage palliation of hypoplastic left heart syndrome. J Thorac Cardiovasc Surg 2003; **126**: 504–9.

Akinturk H, Michel-Benhnke I, Valeskek K et al. Hybrid transcatheter surgical palliation, a basis for univentricular or biventricular repair: the Giessen experience. *Pediatr Cardiol* 2007; **28**: 79–87.

Ohye RG, Sleeper LA, Mahoney L et al. Comparison of shunt types in the Norwood procedure for single ventricle lesions. *N Engl J Med* 2010; **362**: 1980–92.

Cavo-pulmonary Shunts and the Fontan Circulation

David J. Barron

Introduction

A truly univentricular heart is virtually unknown. However, there are a wide variety of different conditions in which there is functionally only one ventricle – typically one dominant ventricle with a second vestigial or underdeveloped ventricle. These 'functionally ventricular morphologies' account for 3 to 4 per cent of all congenital heart disease, but because they all usually require a series of palliative procedures to balance the circulation, they account for 15 to 20 per cent of all congenital heart surgeries. The myriad conditions that fall into this category are summarized in Table 21.1, but regardless of the precise morphology, the principles of management are always the same: stabilize the circulation by ensuring unobstructed venous return, unobstructed systemic outflow and a balanced pulmonary-systemic circulation. Many of these principles are discussed in detail in

Table 21.1 The Fontan Circulation Is the Common Pathway for All Conditions with a Functionally Single Ventricle

Dominant *left* ventricle	Dominant *right* ventricle
Tricuspid atresia	Hypoplastic left heart syndrome
Double-inlet left ventricle (DILV)	DORV with mitral atresia
Pulmonary atresia with intact septum	Unbalanced AVSD (dominant right)
Unbalanced AVSD (dominant left)	
Transposition/VSD with small RV	
Indeterminate dominant ventricle	
Left and right isomerism	

Note: The dominant ventricle can be of either left or right morphology, and this table summarizes the commonest conditions in each group.

Chapters 4 and 20 and apply to the neonatal management of all these conditions.

Once the circulation has been stabilized as a neonate, all these hearts converge on a common pathway towards what is referred to as the 'Fontan circulation'. This describes the situation in which the systemic and pulmonary circulations are placed in series, driven by a single 'pump' – in contrast to the normal circulation, in which the systemic and pulmonary circulations are in parallel, driven by two 'pumps'. This ingenious concept enables the single ventricle to support the entire circulation without any mixing of the bloodstreams and so is (in principle) acyanotic and depends on passive venous pressure to drive the cardiac output through the pulmonary vascular bed. Thus, the Fontan circulation is completely dependent on a low pulmonary vascular resistance (PVR) – and all management of the child prior to Fontan completion is to strive towards protecting the pulmonary vascular bed. These procedures and circulations are referred to as 'palliative' in that they do not achieve a fully 'repaired' circulation – nevertheless, they *are* the definitive procedure for that individual and can provide a remarkably good quality of life. Thus, the rather negative connotation of the word 'palliative' in the more commonly used sense of end-of-life care makes this a rather unfortunate description and should be avoided where possible.

The Cavo-pulmonary Shunt

Conversion from the newborn circulation to the Fontan circulation is a gradual process essentially because of the changes that occur within the lung vasculature and somatic growth during the first months and years of life. PVR is systemic at birth and only comes down to adult levels by the age of six months. The microvasculature of the lungs is also not fully developed for several months, and this is why a systemic shunt is required in a newborn to drive pulmonary blood flow.

However, once a child has reached four to six months of age, the PVR has dropped sufficiently that a high-pressure source of blood flow is no longer required. Instead, the SVC blood can be connected directly into the pulmonary arteries – the cavo-pulmonary shunt. This is a passive shunt that depends entirely on a head of pressure in the systemic veins to drive blood through the pulmonary vasculature as continuous, non-pulsatile flow. This has major advantages over the systemic shunt because it does not place a volume load on the circulation, and it also delivers fully deoxygenated blood to the lungs rather than partially deoxygenated blood. Thus, at the time of cavo-pulmonary shunt, any systemic shunt is usually disconnected, thus removing a volume load from the ventricle and allowing it to function at better loading conditions.

Technique. The procedure is named after William Glenn, who described the procedure in the 1950s as an end-to-end connection between the SVC and the right PA (i.e. flow to only one lung). This has been superseded by an end-to-side anastomosis, as shown in Figure 21.1, and referred to as the 'bidirectional Glenn' shunt to emphasize that flow is to both lungs contrary to the historical depiction (Figure 21.1). The procedure is typically performed at four to six months of age via median sternotomy on cardiopulmonary bypass. It is essential that any stenosis or hypoplasia of the central pulmonary arteries is addressed at the same time to optimize flow to the lungs. The azygous vein must be ligated to prevent SVC blood escaping to the lower-pressure system in the lower half of the body. The SVC is disconnected from the heart at the SVC-RA junction, taking care to preserve the sino-atrial (S-A) node. The procedure can usually be performed with the heart beating unless it needs to be combined with any additional intra-cardiac procedures. Generally, any additional source of pulmonary blood flow is interrupted to create optimal loading conditions for the ventricle. However, there are some schools of thought that think it necessary to leave some additional flow (such as flow through a tightly banded PA) in an attempt to delay the need for the completion operation. Monitoring of the SVC pressure is essential as it will naturally rise to overcome the PVR. Pressures of 15 to 18 mmHg are typical, but greater than 20 mmHg may raise concerns that the PVR is too high. Oxygen saturation SaO_2 of 80 to 85 per cent would be expected. Postoperative management is

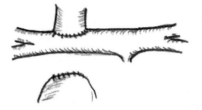

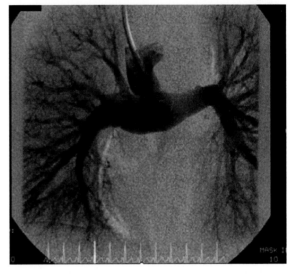

Figure 21.1 The cavo-pulmonary shunt (or bidirectional Glenn shunt).

focused on lowering PVR with oxygen therapy and adequate ventilation. The child should be nursed head up and avoid high positive end-expiratory pressure (PEEP). The procedure is generally low risk, with a 2 to 3 per cent operative mortality, most of which is related to poor underlying ventricular function or high PVR.

Patients with bilateral SVCs will require bilateral anastomoses. Heparin is not usually required unless additional patchwork has had to be placed in the pulmonary arteries. The bidirectional Glenn shunt is a remarkably safe procedure and can be used in a variety of other unusual situations, such as patients with a borderline-sized RV or occasionally even in older patients with a failing and volume-loaded RV, as can occur with untreated Ebstein's anomaly of the tricuspid valve. A natural late consequence of the cavo-pulmonary shunt is the development of arterio-venous fistulae within the lungs, leading to an intra-pulmonary shunt and desaturation. These A-V fistulae appear to be related to a lack of 'hepatic factor' in the blood entering the lungs. As soon as hepatic blood is added to the inflow (such as at completion of the Fontan), the A-V fistulae regress.

Total Cavo-pulmonary Connection

The Fontan circulation is completed by routing the IVC blood flow directly into the lungs such that all the systemic venous blood now 'bypasses' the heart completely (Figure 21.2), hence the name 'total cavo-pulmonary connection' (TCPC). The procedure has almost always been preceded by a bidirectional Glenn shunt, although both connections can be made at the same time in rare cases. This can be achieved in one of two ways:

1. By creating a baffle within the lateral part of the right atrium and connecting the right appendage to the underside of the pulmonary artery. This is referred to as the 'lateral tunnel TCPC'.

2. By separating the IVC from the heart and connecting it to the underside of the pulmonary artery with an external conduit, usually a Gore-Tex tube graft. This is the most commonly used technique and is referred to as the 'extra-cardiac TCPC' (see Table 21.2).

The name derives from the original procedure first performed in 1967 by Francis Fontan in the setting of tricuspid atresia, in which there was no previous bidirectional Glenn and the atrium was connected directly to the pulmonary artery with a homograft conduit. This is now referred to as the 'atrio-pulmonary connection' to differentiate it from the more modern modifications that connect the caval return separately into the PAs.

The procedure will significantly increase pulmonary blood flow, which, again, has to be a passive process driven by the systemic venous pressure. Thus, just as with the bidirectional Glenn, success is entirely dependent on low PVR and well-developed pulmonary arteries. The result of the procedure is that the patient will become fully saturated, but the cost of this is a sudden rise in systemic venous pressure throughout the body. In the immediate postoperative situation, this is not always well tolerated as blood tends to pool within the capacitance of the systemic veins leading to under-filling of the systemic ventricle and low cardiac output. One way of reducing this effect is to create a small fenestration between the

Table 21.2 Comparison of Lateral Tunnel versus Extra-cardiac Total Cavo-pulmonary Connection (TCPC)

	Lateral tunnel	Extra-cardiac
First described:	1988	1998
Bypass technique:	Cross-clamp required	No cross-clamp, no ischaemic time
Fenestration:	Easier and more reliable	Less reliable (commonly closes off)
Right atrium:	Part remains in the Fontan circulation (i.e. at high pressure)	Completely excluded from the Fontan circulation
Atrial arrhythmias:	Commoner	Less common
Age at surgery:	From 18 months	4–5 years

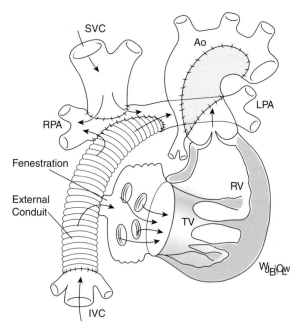

Figure 21.2 The Extra-Cardiac Total Cavo-Pulmonary Connection (TCPC). The IVC is disconnected from the right atrium and connected to the underside of the pulmonary arteries with a prosthetic tube. A small fenestration is made between the conduit and the right atrium . In this example the underlying condition is Hypoplastic Left Heart syndrome but the TCPC can be applied to any functionally univentricular circulation.

Fontan circuit and the pulmonary venous atrium: this allows some blood to escape directly back into the systemic ventricle and so secures better cardiac preload. This creates a small right-to-left shunt and means that SaO_2 tends to drop to the low 90s but is a safer way to manage the circulation. If the fenestration is no longer needed, it can be closed at a later date with a device in the catheterization laboratory. The second immediate consequence of the raised systemic venous pressure is an increased resistance to lymphatic return, resulting in the build-up of tissue oedema and fluid collection in the 'third space', particularly the pleural cavities.

Technique. Definitive imaging of the pulmonary arteries and measurement of PA pressure and transpulmonary gradient are essential. In bicaval cannulation, cannulate the IVC as low as possible. A lateral tunnel TCPC requires application of a cross-clamp, the right atrium is opened widely and a separate incision is made into the underside of the right PA. The right atrial appendage is opened and anastomosed to this opening, augmenting with a patch anteriorly if necessary. A baffle (usually Gore-Tex) is then placed into the atrium to separate it into two components – the lateral tunnel carrying the IVC blood up through to the pulmonary arteries. A simple fenestration (usually 5 to 6 mm) is punched into the Gore-Tex baffle, and the right atrium is closed. It is important to place a pressure monitoring line into the pulmonary venous atrium so that the preload on the ventricle can be monitored postoperatively.

The extra-cardiac TCPC can be performed without need for a cross-clamp. The IVC is disconnected from the heart with a side-biting clamp across the distal right atrium (thus the importance of mobilizing the IVC extensively and cannulating very inferiorly). An opening is made in the underside of the right PA, and a Gore-Tex tube graft is interposed between this opening and the IVC. A fenestration is created by punching a hole in the medial side of the Gore-Tex graft and an opening into the facing side of the right atrial appendage – the two are then anastomosed using side-biting clamps (Figure 21.2).

Postoperative care is focused on providing adequate preload (hence the importance of having a left atrial pressure line), and patients may need considerable volume replacement due to the capacitance effect of blood pooling in the venous reservoir, together with early extubation where possible – positive-pressure ventilation will significantly reduce cardiac

output because all flow into the lungs is completely dependent on passive flow at low pressure. Patients are fully anti-coagulated due to the risk of clot forming on the Gore-Tex surface, and chest drains need to remain in situ for several days until the pleural drainage has settled. Operative mortality is 3 to 4 per cent, and outcome is strongly influenced by two key factors that define success for the Fontan circulation: low PVR and well-reserved ventricular function.

The timing for TCPC varies according to institutional preference and is generally performed between 18 months and five years of age. The extra-cardiac conduit must use a conduit that will carry the adult-calibre IVC, so it tends to be delayed, where possible, until the child has reached an age at which at least a 16- to 18-mm tube can be accommodated (typically four years of age).

Further Reading

Alsoufi B, Manlhiot C, Awan A et al. Current outcomes of the Glenn bidirectional cavopulmonary connection for single ventricle palliation. *Eur J Cardiothorac Surg* 2012; **42**(1): 42–48.

Azakie A, McCrindle BW, Van Arsdell G et al. Extracardiac conduit versus lateral tunnel cavopulmonary connections at a single institution: impact on outcomes. *J Thorac Cardiovasc Surg* 2001; **122**(6): 1219–28.

de Leval MR. Evolution of the Fontan-Kreutzer procedure. *Semin Thorac Cardiovasc Surg Pediatr Card Surg Annu* 2010; **13**: 91–95.

de Leval MR, Kilner P, Gewillig M, Bull C. Total cavopulmonary connection: a logical alternative to atriopulmonary connection for complex Fontan operations. Experimental studies and early clinical experience. *J Thorac Cardiovasc Surg* 1988; **96**(5): 682–95.

d'Udekem Y, Iyengar AJ, Cochrane AD et al. The Fontan procedure: contemporary techniques have improved long-term outcomes. *Circulation* 2007; **116**: 157–74.

Fontan F, Baudet E. Surgical repair of tricuspid atresia. *Thorax* 1971; **26**: 240–48.

Fontan F, Kirklin JW, Fernandez G et al. Outcome after a 'perfect' Fontan operation. *Circulation* 1990; **81**(5): 1520–36.

Gérelli S, Boulitrop C, Van Steenberghe M et al. Bidirectional cavopulmonary shunt with additional pulmonary blood flow: a failed or successful strategy? *Eur J Cardiothorac Surg* 2012; **42**(3): 513–19.

Hosein RB, Clarke AJ, McGuirk SP et al. Factors influencing early and late outcome following the Fontan procedure in the current era: the 'two commandments'? *Eur J Cardiothorac Surg* 2007; **31**(3): 344–52.

Kreutzer G, Galindez E, Bono H. An operation for the correction of tricuspid atresia. *J Thorac Cardiovasc Surg* 1973; **66**: 613–21

Marcelletti C, Corno A, Giannico S, Marino B. Inferior vena cava-pulmonary artery extracardiac conduit. A new form of right heart bypass. *J Thorac Cardiovasc Surg* 1990; **100**: 228–32.

Robbers-Visser D, Miedema M, Nijveld A et al. Results of staged total cavopulmonary connection for functionally univentricular hearts; comparison of intra-atrial lateral tunnel and extracardiac conduit. *Eur J Cardiothorac Surg* 2010; **37**(4): 934–41.

Rogers LS, Glatz AC, Ravishankar C et al. Eighteen years of the Fontan operation at a single institution: results from 771 consecutive patients. *J Am Coll Cardiol* 2012; **60**: 1018–25.

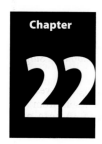

Chapter

22

Vascular Rings

David J. Barron

Introduction

Vascular rings are a group of rare congenital abnormalities in which the great vessels form a complete ring of vascular structure around the trachea and oesophagus. Most are due to the persistence of embryological structures, often in combination with abnormal vascular patterns.

They do not cause cardiovascular symptoms. Their clinical significance and management are entirely related to the compression they cause to the trachea and oesophagus. If they cause no compression, then they do not require treatment.

There are three main types of vascular rings:

1. **Double Aortic Arch.** Commonest variety, accounting for 40 to 50 per cent of cases. This is caused by persistence of the embryological fourth arch causing a complete ring around the trachea and oesophagus (Figures 22.1 and 22.2). Each arch gives rise to a carotid and subclavian artery, and the descending thoracic aorta usually then adopts a normal course down the leftward side of the vertebral columns. Thus, the right arch has to pass behind the oesophagus (creating the characteristic posterior indentation on barium swallow) to reach the left side. Both arches can be of equal size, but the commonest pattern is for the right arch to be dominant – the left side is typically hypoplastic or even atretic (i.e. a fibrous cord) beyond the subclavian origin. It is very rare (almost unknown) for the left arch to be dominant. The ductal ligament will run into the posterior aspect of the arch, creating a second component to the ring.

2. **Right Aortic Arch with Left Ductus.** This is the second commonest (25 to 30 per cent) and occurs when the arch is right sided (i.e. passes over the right main bronchus) but reverts back to the left side at the descending aorta, where the ductus ligament inserts into it (Figures 22.3 and 22.4). Although the head and neck vessels can arise normally, the commonest arrangement in a vascular ring (70 per cent of cases) is for anomalous origin of the left subclavian from the posterior arch, which is also the site of insertion of the ductus ligament. The anomalous subclavian usually arises from a short out-pouching called the 'diverticulum of Kommerell' that represents the persistence of the posterior remnant of the fourth arch. A left arch with right-sided ductus has been reported but is extremely rare.

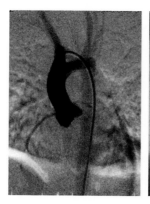
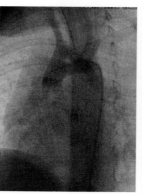
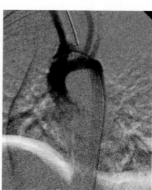

Figure 22.1 Angiogram showing complete double arch. A subclavian and carotid artery arise from each arch.

3. **Left Pulmonary Artery Sling.** This is the third commonest type (15 to 20 per cent) and differs from the other rings in two important ways: firstly, in that the sling passes only around the trachea,

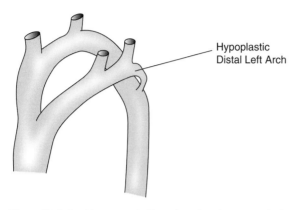

Hypoplastic Distal Left Arch

Figure 22.2 Double aortic arch. The right arch is dominant, which is the commonest arrangement. In this case, the left arch is hypoplastic beyond the origin of the left subclavian artery.

and secondly, the anomaly is strongly associated with varying degrees of tracheal stenosis, including complete tracheal rings (50 to 67 per cent). The sling is created by the aberrant origin of the left PA from the right PA that runs behind the trachea to reach the left hilum (Figure 22.5). The ring is completed by the duct ligament that inserts into the left PA on leftward side of the trachea.

Presentation

Between 50 and 67 per cent of cases present in the first year of life and are most commonly related to tracheal compression causing a stridor or 'noisy breathing'. There may be a history of recurrent chest infections, or the stridor may be picked up on examination during one of these episodes. Younger children may have a characteristic 'seal-bark' cough, and older children may have a chronic non-productive

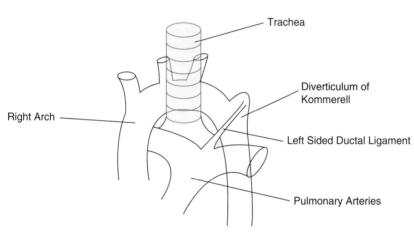

Trachea

Diverticulum of Kommerell

Right Arch

Left Sided Ductal Ligament

Pulmonary Arteries

Figure 22.3 Right aortic arch with left-sided ductus ligament. The trachea and oesophagus are trapped in the ring.

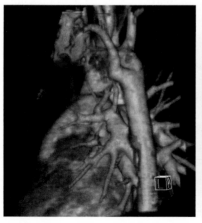

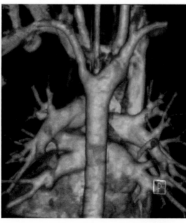

Figure 22.4 MRI reconstruction showing a right-sided arch with anomalous left subclavian artery arising from a diverticulum of Kommerell. The ductal ligament will insert into the base of the diverticulum but does not show on the MRI. (A black-and-white version of this figure will appear in some formats. For the colour version, please refer to the plate section.)

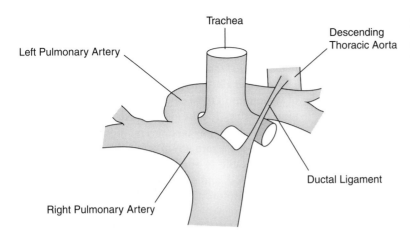

Figure 22.5 Pulmonary artery sling: The left pulmonary artery arises as the first branch of the right pulmonary artery, encircling the trachea.

cough due to tracheal irritation or have been mis-diagnosed as 'asthmatic'. Severity of symptoms is variable, but generally, the more severe the compression, the earlier is the presentation. The stridor is not only due to the compression but also due to a degree of tracheo-broncho-malacia of the affected segment of the airway.

Oesophageal symptoms are less severe, but there may be a history of dysphagia. Infants may have been noticed to have frequent vomiting or drooling of saliva. However, the dysphagia is not usually severe enough to prevent normal nutrition or cause failure to thrive.

Diagnosis and Investigation

Clinical examination may reveal stridor, and there may be signs of lobar collapse and consolidation. CXR is not usually diagnostic but may show hyperinflation due to air trapping or localized signs of collapse/consolidation. The mediastinal shadow may show the characteristic knuckle of a double arch or suggest a right-sided arch.

Barium swallow is very helpful for diagnosis and shows a characteristic fixed posterior indentation (that is pulsatile on screening) which represents the right-sided arch passing posteriorly. In pulmonary artery sling, the indentation will be anterior. Although diagnostic, this does not give anatomical information on the nature of the ring, and CT scan or MRI is required for definitive investigation – defining the position of the arch and head and neck vessels. Atretic segments (fibrous cords or ductal ligaments) cannot always be seen, but the anatomical pattern of the vessels together with evidence of localized tracheal compression will

confirm the diagnosis. Echocardiography is helpful, particularly in pulmonary artery sling, but angiography is not usually necessary.

Formal airway assessment is not usually necessary except in the case of PA sling, where it is essential due to the common association with tracheal anomalies.

Management

Treatment is based on severity of symptoms. Mild symptoms can be managed conservatively with reassurance and dietary advice, but any evidence of significant airway obstruction will require surgical release with or without a procedure to overcome any tracheomalacia (aortopexy or tracheopexy).

Surgery requires careful planning and thorough investigation to delineate the anatomy. Most can be approached via a postero-lateral thoracotomy in the fourth space. A left-sided approach is used in the vast majority of cases – except in the case of double arch with a dominant left arch, which is extremely rare. In double arch, the approach is on the side of the non-dominant arch, which is divided beyond the origin of the subclavian artery, and the ductal ligament is also divided. In the unusual case of equal-sized arches, the approach should be on the side of the descending aorta as this will provide access to the site of duct insertion (again, usually the left side). If there is any doubt over the dominance of the, arch or if there are other intra-cardiac lesions requiring surgery at the same time, then a midline sternotomy approach should be used. Each arch can be test occluded with a clamp in turn, and any changes in the femoral blood pressure can be recorded to help identify which arch is to be safely divided.

There is frequently a clear release of tension as the ring is divided. The distal end tends to fall away behind the oesophagus, being pulled away by the rightward arch. It is therefore very important that secure haemostasis of the distal end is achieved before removing the side-biting clamp on the vessel and also important that a vascular sling has been placed around the distal right arch so that it can be retrieved if there is any bleeding.

A right-sided arch with left duct is also dealt with via a left thoracotomy. An aberrant left subclavian artery does not usually need further attention after the ring has been divided. However, some authors recommend division of the artery (and Kommerell's diverticulum, if present) and re-implantation into the side of the left common carotid artery using side-biting clamps on the vessels.

PA sling is best managed via a midline sternotomy. Both pulmonary arteries are fully mobilized, chasing the left PA behind the trachea and identifying it where it reappears on the leftward side. The duct ligament is divided. A side-biting clamp is placed on the origin of the left PA, which is then divided, the defect in the right PA being directly over-sewn. The clamp can then be removed from the right PA, and the left PA is flipped out from behind the trachea and brought forward to lie next to the main PA. A side-biting clamp is then placed on the leftward side of the main PA, and a vertical incision is made to receive the left PA. This is most safely done using cardiopulmonary bypass, although it can be done without.

If there is associated tracheal stenosis/hypoplasia associated with the PA sling, this may require surgical repair at the same time. Localized stenoses can be treated with resection and direct reanastomosis or with sliding tracheoplasty for longer stenoses. More extensive stenoses (often with complete tracheal rings) require extensive tracheal reconstruction on cardiopulmonary bypass and should only be undertaken by specialist teams. It is important that the tracheal anatomy is accurately assessed preoperatively so that patients who need tracheal reconstruction can be referred to specialist centres – surgery to the PA sling may interfere with the tissue planes around the trachea and jeopardize tracheal vascularity, making a reoperation much more difficult; thus, it is very important that both are dealt with simultaneously.

Outcomes. Surgery is safe and carries a risk of 1 to 2 per cent, except in the case of associated tracheal stenosis, where the risk can be much higher in neonates with extensive stenoses (in-hospital mortality of 15 to 20 per cent). There is immediate improvement of symptoms in most cases, but complete resolution is unusual due to the associated tracheo-bronchomalacia, which may take several months to resolve.

These are a rare group of conditions but are eminently suitable to surgical repair. Long-term results are very good, and patients should expect permanent relief of symptoms. The complex tracheal reconstruction group remains the greatest challenge, and prognosis depends on this rather than on the underlying vascular ring. Late aneurysms of Kommerell's diverticulum have been described, which supports the practice of aiming to resent as much of the diverticulum as possible at the time of initial repair.

The condition has benefitted from the development of new imaging modalities of high-definition CT and MRI. Recognition of the importance of co-existing tracheomalacia has led to a more thorough approach to assessing the airway preoperatively. Both preoperative and intra-operative bronchoscopy are likely to become commoner in the management of these patients, just as video-assisted thoracoscopic (VATS) surgery is likely to be more widely applied to the more straightforward surgical repairs.

Concomitant tracheomalacia can be difficult to assess. In general, division of the vascular ring alone will relieve the symptoms. However, the more severe the compression and the younger the patient, the greater is the likelihood of significant secondary tracheomalacia. This is why we recommend performing bronchoscopy at the time of surgery to assess the trachea before and after division of the ring. If there is significant tracheomalacia, then there are two surgical options. The first is aortopexy, in which the ascending aorta is brought forward towards the back of the sternum with a double-armed pledgetted suture placed through the aortic adventia. This can be performed through the same thoracotomy incision or through a separate anterior mediastinotomy in the second intercostal space. It is important that the fascial attachments between the aorta and the trachea are left intact so that the manoeuvre opens up the anterior trachea. The second option is seen in patients in whom a midline sternotomy is used, in which case a tracheopexy can be performed in a similar way.

The trachea is mobilized along the malacic segment, and pledgetted sutures are placed in the anterior wall on the left and right sides through a tracheal cartilaginous ring. These sutures are then suspended (tied) to the back of the sternum at the sterno-chondral junctions to help splint open the trachea.

Further Reading

Antón-Pacheco JL, Cano I, Comas J et al. Management of congenital tracheal stenosis in infancy. *Eur J Cardiothorac Surg* 2006; **29**: 991–96.

Backer CL, Ilbawi MN, Idriss FS, De Leon SY. Vascular anomalies causing tracheoesophageal compression: review of experience in children. *J Thorac Cardiovasc Surg* 1989; **97**: 725–31.

Backer Cl, Mavroudis C, Holinger LD. Repair of congenital tracheal stenosis. *Semin Thorac Cadiovasc Surg Paediatr Card Surg Annu* 2002; **5**: 173–86.

Backer CL, Mavroudis C, Rigsby CK, Holinger LD. Trends in vascular ring surgery. *J Thorac Cardiovasc Surg* 2005; **129**: 1339–47.

Bonnard A, Auber F, Fourcade L et al. Vascular ring abnormalities: a retrospective study of 62 cases. *J Pediatr Surg* 2003; **38**: 539–43.

Fiore AC, Brown JW, Weber TR, Turrentine MW. Surgical treatment of pulmonary artery sling and tracheal stenosis. *Ann Thorac Surg* 2005; **79**: 38–46.

Grillo HC, Wright CD, Vlahakes GJ, MacGillvray TE. Management of congenital tracheal stenosis by means of slide tracheoplasty or resection and reconstruction, with long-term follow up of growth after slide tracheoplasty. *J Thorac Cardiovasc Surg* 2002; **123**: 145–52.

Haramati LB, Glickstein JS, Issenberg HJ, Haramati N, Crooke GA. MR imaging and CT of vascular anomalies and connections in patients with congenital heart disease: significance in surgical planning.. *Radiographics* 2002; **22**: 337–47.

Linna O, Hyrynkangas K, Lanning P, Niemenan P. Central airways stenosis in school-aged children: differential diagnosis from asthma. *Acta Paediatr* 2002; **91**: 399–402.

Chapter 23

Hybrid Cardiac Surgical Procedures in Congenital Heart Disease

Oliver Stumper

Introduction

A great number of congenital cardiac lesions are now being treated by interventional cardiac catheterization techniques. Advances in equipment and devices have allowed for trans-catheter closure of some 75 per cent of all secundum atrial septal defects (ASDs), virtually all cases of patent arterial duct in childhood (except premature neonates) and a fair number of ventricular septal defects (VSDs) in older children. Further, virtually all cases of pulmonary valve stenosis and a large number of aortic valve stenoses from neonates to young adults are being treated by catheter balloon valvuloplasty. Intravascular stent designs have evolved and have proved highly effective in enlarging pulmonary arterial vessels, which may not be easily accessible to a cardiac surgical approach. Treatment of adolescent and adult native or re-coarctation is now virtually entirely catheter based. The development of trans-catheter devices is rapidly progressing – in the future, biodegradable devices will become commonplace, thereby further expanding the indication for trans-catheter treatment.

Cardiopulmonary bypass in itself carries mortality and morbidity. Increasingly, cardiac surgeons and interventional cardiologists work together to develop ways of treatment to make bypass times shorter and achieve highly successful patient outcomes at reduced risk. This so-called hybrid approach is evolving and is destined to become one of the major treatment avenues for congenital heart disease in the future. As these techniques become more commonplace and the availability of specifically designed hybrid cardiac theatres increases, there is likely to be a future training demand for cardiac surgeons to develop some of the wire skills required for cardiac catheter work. At the same time, there is a need to refine existing catheter equipment and to develop bespoke equipment to maximize on the true potential of these techniques (Figure 23.1).

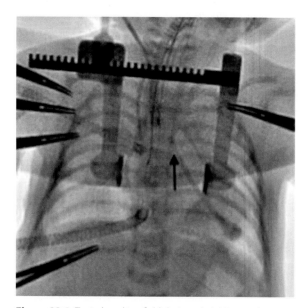

Figure 23.1 Typical working field during a hybrid procedure in a 3-kg neonate. The tip of the sheath (arrow) is placed in the main pulmonary artery and is secured by a purse-string suture. Access is limited not only by the bypass cannulae and the sternal spreader but also by the X-ray tube some 10 cm above the surgical field.

Exit Angiography. The routine use of intra-operative epicardial or trans-oesophageal ultrasound techniques has been established for more than two decades in surgery for congenital heart disease. However, ultrasound techniques are limited with regards to assessment of reconstructed pulmonary arteries and the aortic arch.

In the majority of patients after complex pulmonary artery reconstruction or unifocalization procedures, it is of value to assess the surgical results immediately after weaning off bypass in order to check on the integrity of the repair and the morphology of the reconstructed pulmonary arteries and obtain central pulmonary arterial pressures. At the end of the bypass run, the X-ray tube is moved into position. The right atrium or main pulmonary artery is punctured with a needle, and a 0.018-inch wire is placed, over which a No. 4 French short introducer sheath is inserted. The dilator sheath is removed, blood is aspirated, and pressures are transduced. A single dose of diluted contrast agent (0.5–1 mL/kg of body weight) is injected rapidly either manually or by pump whilst acquiring the images either at 15 or 30 frames per second. The passage through the lungs and the capillary bed is recorded and can be reviewed on the video monitors for detailed analysis. If significant narrowing of the reconstructed pulmonary arteries is identified, there must be a discussion as to whether (1) to accept the result for the time being, (2) whether to revise the observed lesion surgically or (3) whether to consider stent implantation. Balloon angioplasty for postsurgical strictures immediately after bypass is unsafe and probably ineffective. Stenting of such lesions is safer and allows one to straighten out any observed kinks. Running polypropylene sutures can safely be over-dilated to some 20 per cent.

Post-Bypass Atrial Septal Stenting. In some cases, filling pressures after weaning from bypass may be excessively high after complete closure of an ASD. In such cases, a small atrial communication may be of benefit for early postoperative recovery. The right atrium can be punctured under direct vision, and the needle can be advanced under epicardial ultrasound guidance into the left atrium. A wire is introduced to the left atrium, and a No. 4 or 5 French short sheath is placed within the left atrium. A test injection is conducted to delineate the plane of the atrial septum under 30- to 40-degree left anterior oblique angiographic projection. A balloon catheter is then advanced across the atrial septum and inflated fully. The resultant communication will normally measure about half the chosen balloon diameter and is unlikely to remain open for a long time. More reliable communications can be created by placing a premounted coronary or renal stent. The stent is advanced across the atrial septum. The introducer sheath is withdrawn to the right atrial side, still covering part of the stent, and the balloon is inflated, to achieve flaring of the left atrial side. The sheath is then withdrawn well into the right atrial cavity. The balloon is inflated further so as to dilate the right atrial aspect of the stent to achieve a diablo configuration.

Peri-ventricular Device Closure of VSD. The majority of muscular VSDs close spontaneously during the first six to 12 months of life. However, if a significant defect/shunt persists after six months of age, there may be a need for intervention. In cases with multiple defects and in the presence of cardiac failure, pulmonary artery (PA) banding may be indicated. However, peri-ventricular closure of the largest VSDs may be the better option.

After (limited) median sternotomy, the right ventricular cavity is entered by a needle, and an appropriately sized guide wire and sheath are advanced across the defect straight into the left ventricular cavity under ultrasound control (either direct epicardial or trans-oesophageal). Defect dimensions are measured in at least two planes during diastole, and an appropriately sized short sheath is selected. The device is placed under ultrasound control. Repeat angiography through the left atrial appendage with left anterior oblique and cranial angulation may be indicated to identify and plan closure of additional defects.

The same techniques can be employed after surgical correction of congenital heart disease when the post-bypass cardiac ultrasound study documents persistence of a residual muscular VSD.

Peri-ventricular Stenting of the Systemic Ductus. The surgical management of hypoplastic left heart syndrome (HLHS) is based around the Norwood procedure and its modifications (see Chapter 20). Over the past 10 years, an alternative strategy for initial management has evolved that avoids the need for bypass surgery using hybrid techniques: bilateral pulmonary artery bands are placed to control pulmonary blood flow, the duct is stented open and the atrial septum is stretched open. This is now referred to as the 'hybrid Norwood procedure' for the treatment of HLHS. Via a median sternotomy, the individual pulmonary arteries are banded using a short length of 3- to 3.5-mm Gore-Tex shunt. Next, the main pulmonary artery is punctured with a needle, and a short introducer sheath is placed within the main pulmonary artery (Figure 23.2). It is important to choose a stent to cover the entire length of the ductus without compromising retrograde flow to the ascending aorta, in particular, in patients with aortic coarctation. The sheath is then advanced across the ductus arteriosus into the descending aorta. A balloon or self-expandable stent is used to stent the ductus under fluoroscopic guidance (Figure 23.3). Finally, any restriction across the atrial septum is relieved by static or pull-back septostomy from a separate puncture of the right atrial free wall. Alternatively, a stent can be placed across the atrial septum (see earlier).

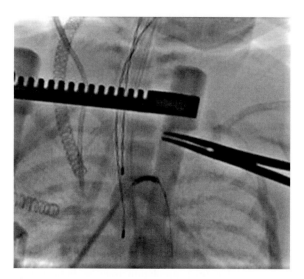

Figure 23.2 Left anterior oblique projection of the ductus arteriosus during hybrid stenting. Sidearm contrast injections are being used to define the anatomy of the duct and the ideal position for stent placement. Landmarks during placement of the stent include the various radio-opaque objects such as the nasogastric tube and thermistor.

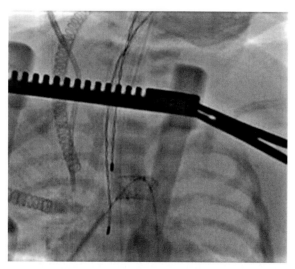

Figure 23.3 Fully deployed stent. Repeat angiography is performed to exclude retro-aortic obstruction and encroachment of the stent on the branch pulmonary arteries.

Some centres have reported excellent results with such an approach, but most reserve this approach for high-risk cases in which avoidance of cardiopulmonary bypass is an advantage (<2.5 kg in body weight, haemodynamic instability, cerebral or intestinal bleeding).

Concerns remain over the applicability of this approach in children with coarctation of the aorta, in whom there may result a strict limitation to retrograde coronary artery supply and over the increased afterload of pulmonary artery bands and the stented duct in parallel. Nonetheless, banding of the pulmonary arteries in compromised children with HLHS has proven to be a good staging therapy for acute management. In some of these children, maintained on prostaglandin infusion, stenting of the arterial duct either from a trans-femoral route or from a periventricular route may be the right approach – in others, conversion to a standard first-stage surgical Norwood procedure may be the better option. Comparative and, importantly, randomized trials are under way and urgently needed to define the role of this novel hybrid approach to an established surgical approach.

Intra-operative Stenting of Pulmonary Arteries.
Surgical pulmonary artery repair most frequently involves patch augmentation of stenosed segments. However, surgical reconstruction may be limited by external compression (such as after a Damus/Norwood connection) or if lesions are within the hilum. In these cases, an interventional catheter approach may be more rewarding. In cases with external compression, the insertion of an endovascular stent is highly effective and limits the time required to dissect out the pulmonary arteries underneath the great arteries (aorta-Damus connection). In a low-pressure pulmonary circulation, such as after a cavopulmonary shunt, our experience is that neointima proliferation after stenting is a rare long-term complication. Thus, in cases with a passive pulmonary circulation (cavo-pulmonary shunt or Fontan), stenting of central pulmonary arteries has become our preferred technique. In these cases, cardiac surgical intervention (extra-cardiac Fontan connection) is completed first; then a pulmonary angiogram is performed via a directly inserted sheath within the pulmonary artery pathways. The narrowed pulmonary artery is intubated with a diagnostic catheter directly, and a guide wire is placed into a distal segment. A stent with potential for further expansion is selected and placed across the area of narrowing, sparing the upper-lobe segment of the branch pulmonary artery. The stent is dilated to greater than the predicted size of the branch pulmonary artery. Ideally, this should also cover the anastomosis, and the proximal end should be flared.

In selected cases it may be better to implant a stent directly under surgical vision and to flare the proximal end. In this setting, the stent may be further secured by placing some stitches through the struts of the stent. However, when using this technique of stent placement under direct vision, great care has to be taken that the stent does not impinge on the first distal branches of the vessel, which cannot be adequately visualized throughout the procedure.

Pulmonary Balloon Dilatation. In selected children with tetralogy of Fallot who have a pulmonary valve annulus of some −2 to −5 Z-scores, there may be the option to perform balloon dilatation of the pulmonary valve as an alternative to trans-annular patching with a mono-cusp patch. The balloon chosen should measure some 1.3 to 1.5 times the size of the pulmonary valve annulus. Balloon length should not exceed 2 cm. The balloon is inflated manually under fluoroscopic control or using a pressure-controlled inflation device to nominal working pressure (typically some 6 to 8 atm). Initial reports suggest that the incidence of trans-annular patching in the surgical correction of tetralogy of Fallot can be reduced by this technique, which in turn may reduce the need for late pulmonary valve implantation for progressive right ventricular dilatation.

Peri-ventricular Valve Implantation. For many years the trans-apical implantation of trans-catheter aortic valves from a limited sternotomy has been a high-volume hybrid procedure with very encouraging results in high-risk adults. At the same time, with further miniaturization of the catheter equipment, there will be a greater use of the percutaneous approach other than for patients with very significant peripheral arterial disease. Soon trans-catheter valves will become available that can be placed effectively through Nos. 14 to 16 French catheters (rather than the current Nos. 24 to 26 French sheaths). A further development will be the peri-ventricular implantation of pulmonary valves in the growing adult population after Fallot repair with free pulmonary regurgitation

and right ventricular dilatation. Self-expanding valve frameworks are most likely to cater for the large variation of outflow tract morphology observed in these patients.

The hybrid approach to the treatment of congenital heart disease is a relatively recent technique that offers great opportunities to further the cooperation between cardiac surgeons and interventional cardiologists. This undoubtedly will result in modification of the approaches and current techniques used in the treatment of congenital heart disease. Future theatre installations and training programmes both in cardiac surgery and in interventional cardiology have to recognize this trend and make appropriate adjustments to achieve maximum impact and patient benefit.

Further Reading

Akintuerk H, Michael-Behnke I, Valeske K et al. Stenting of the arterial duct and banding of the pulmonary arteries: basis for combined Norwood stage 1 and 2 repair in hypoplastic left heart. *Circulation* 2002; **105**: 1099–103.

Bacha EA, Daves S, Hardin J et al. Single ventricle palliation for high-risk neonates: the emergence of an alternative hybrid stage 1 strategy. *J Thorac Cardiovasc Surg* 2006; **131**: 163–71.

Galantowicz M, Cheatham JP. Lessons learned from the development of a new hybrid strategy for the management of hypoplastic left heart syndrome. *Pediatr Cardiol* 2005; **26**: 190–99.

Holzer RJ, Sisk M, Chisolm JL et al. Completion angiography after cardiac surgery for congenital heart disease: complementing the intraoperative imaging modalities. *Pediatr Cardiol* 2009; **30**(8): 1075–82.

Michel-Behnke I, Ewert P, Koch A et al. Device closure of ventricular septal defects by hybrid procedures: a multicenter retrospective study. *Catheter Cardiovasc Intervent* 2011; **77**(2): 242–51.

Vida VL, Padalino MA, Maschietto N et al. The balloon dilation of the pulmonary valve during early repair of tetralogy of Fallot. *Catheter Cardiovasc Intervent* 2012; **80**(6): 915–21.

Extra-corporeal Membrane Oxygenation in Children

Timothy J. Jones

Introduction

Extra-corporeal membrane oxygenation (ECMO) is a technique of providing total cardiac and/or respiratory support. It uses an extra-corporeal circuit similar to cardiopulmonary bypass. It remains the mainstay of short-term mechanical circulatory support in neonates, infants and children with cardiac and/or respiratory failure.

The two commonest modes of ECMO support are

- *Veno-venous ECMO*, which provides respiratory support only. Blood is drained from the venous circulation, oxygenated and returned to the venous circulation (VVECMO). In VVECMO, no direct cardiac support is provided.
- *Veno-arterial ECMO*, which provides cardiac and respiratory support. Blood is drained from the venous circulation, oxygenated and returned to the arterial circulation, thereby bypassing the heart and lungs (VAECMO).

The most frequent indication for ECMO remains the treatment of neonatal respiratory failure secondary to aetiologies such as persistent pulmonary hypertension of the newborn (PPHN), meconium aspiration, sepsis, respiratory distress syndrome and congenital diaphragmatic hernia (CDH). Internationally, there is an increasing use of ECMO in children with myocardial failure following cardiac surgery or as a consequence of myocarditis or cardiomyopathy.

The aim of support is to provide adequate oxygenation and preservation of end-organ function to allow time for either myocardial recovery ('bridge to recovery') or as temporary support before converting to longer-term support such as a ventricular assist device (VAD) ('bridge to bridge') or as support to transplantation ('bridge to transplant').

Data from the Extracorporeal Life Support Organisation (ELSO) 2012 international registry reports an overall survival rate to discharge for neonates and children of 68.5 per cent following ECMO. The best survival rates are seen in neonates and children following respiratory ECMO of 75 and 56 per cent, respectively. The survival to discharge following ECMO for cardiac support is 40 per cent in neonates and 49 per cent in children.

Indications

ECMO should be considered in patients with circulatory and/or respiratory failure that is refractory to maximal conventional treatment, providing that the underlying disease process is potentially reversible and that they do not have an absolute contra-indication.

In respiratory failure, the oxygen index (OI) can be used to assess the severity of the illness. An OI greater than 25 is associated with a mortality of 25 per cent with conventional respiratory support, and the mortality rises to 80 per cent with an OI of over 40.

$$\text{Oxygen index} = \frac{\text{FiO}_2 \times \text{mean airway pressure}}{\text{PaO}_2}$$

An OI in excess of 40 is usually an indicator for the need for respiratory ECMO. However, the OI must be assessed as part of the overall condition of the child and his or her response to treatment. An OI of 43 that rapidly falls in response to high-frequency oscillation ventilation or nitric oxide is not necessarily an indication for ECMO in contrast to an OI of over 30 that gradually climbs regardless of all therapeutic interventions.

There is no equivalent to OI for cardiac support. VAECMO should be considered in patients preoperatively who either cannot be stabilized prior to corrective surgery or are in low cardiac output that is either thought to be recoverable or as a bridge to cardiac transplantation. Increasingly, following cardiac surgery, ECMO is being used in patients who cannot be separated from cardiopulmonary bypass or in whom there is refractory low cardiac output postoperatively. There is also an increasing use of ECMO following cardiac arrest (ECPR), but in most institutions this is limited to patients following cardiac surgery or during a witnessed cardiac arrest in hospital. The indicators for cardiac support are those of persistent low cardiac output such as persistent metabolic acidosis, high inotropic requirement, hypotension and oliguria in the setting of myocardial failure or dysrhythmias.

Contra-indications. Brain death and irreversible multi-organ dysfunction are clear contra-indications to ECMO. Prolonged anti-coagulation and severely reduced long-term functional ability are similarly contra-indications. A corrected gestational age of less than 34 weeks is associated with a significant increase in morbidity and mortality, as well as presenting problems with cannulation and management and consequently is a contra-indication. Previously, prolonged mechanical ventilation at high pressure for greater than 10 days was a contra-indication, but this is increasingly becoming only a relative contra-indication.

Equipment

All ECMO circuits consist of cannulae, a membrane oxygenator, heat exchanger and blood pump all connected by PVC tubing. Cannulation in neonates is usually via the neck vessels (right internal jugular vein and common carotid artery) or centrally via a sternotomy using the right atrium and aorta. In older children or adults, the femoral vessels are proportionally larger and may be used for cannulation.

In VVECMO, a specifically designed dual-lumen cannula may be placed via the right internal jugular vein with the tip sitting low in the right atrium. The cannula is designed to facilitate venous drainage proximally via one lumen with return of oxygenated blood distally via the second lumen to the right atrium in an attempt to reduce the recirculation of re-infused oxygenated blood around the ECMO circuit. Alternatively, or in addition, another cannula may be placed via the femoral vein for venous drainage with return of oxygenated blood via the internal jugular vein.

In recent years, due to evolving blood pump technology, there has been a move away from using roller pumps for flow generation with an increasing use of centrifugal pumps. These pumps are non-occlusive and preload and afterload dependent, so a flow probe must always be used because blood flow is not directly proportional to pump speed. Blood flow is also influenced by the volume status of the patient and his or her systemic vascular resistance as well as resistances that may exist or develop in the circuit. Centrifugal pumps develop a significant negative pressure on their inlet side that can aid with venous drainage. These factors mean that it is not necessary to incorporate a venous bladder or capacitance in the circuit, as is the case when using a roller pump. It has also meant that transporting the patient on ECMO has become easier with venous drainage less dependent on gravity.

In supporting patients on VAECMO, it is important to ensure that the heart is completely decompressed. Adequate venous drainage usually decompresses the right ventricle, but even with the best drainage, it is only possible to drain approximately 80 per cent of venous return. If there is a significant atrial septal defect (ASD) or ventricular septal defect (VSD), the left ventricle may decompress adequately, but if not, then either an atrial septostomy should be performed or a direct cannula or 'vent' placed via the left atrial appendage or pulmonary vein and connected to the venous drainage line. The left ventricle will be unlikely to recover if it is not adequately decompressed due to suboptimal coronary and subendocardial perfusion. Regular echocardiography must be performed to ensure adequate cardiac decompression, exclude mediastinal collections, confirm cannula position and monitor cardiac function and recovery.

Patients receive systemic anti-coagulation prior to commencement of ECMO and are maintained on a heparin infusion to achieve an activated clotting time (ACT) of 180 to 200 seconds. Bleeding is one of the commonest complications of ECMO, and there is a continual balance required between sufficient anti-coagulation to prevent thrombus and subsequent embolization from the circuit but not excessive to avoid bleeding. Despite adequate anti-coagulation, fibrin will always be deposited throughout the circuit, which must be checked frequently for developing thrombus.

In VVECMO, the adequacy of oxygen delivery can be difficult to ascertain. This is because some of the oxygenated blood delivered to the right atrium will re-circulate around the ECMO circuit, and the amount of re-circulation will be variable. Measuring the venous line saturations may give a falsely elevated number if re-circulation is high. The patient's own lungs will contribute a variable amount to oxygenation, and the cardiac output may be variable depending on cardiac reserve and oxygenation. Determining the adequacy of oxygen delivery relies upon assessing the patient's arterial blood saturations. This should be done in association with assessing the venous drainage line saturations. If the patient's arterial saturations are low, but the venous line saturations are high, this suggests a high amount of re-circulation. Pump flow rates are always reduced to the minimum required to achieve arterial saturations of 70 to 85 per cent. Higher pump flow rates may be associated with increased re-circulation.

In VAECMO, the adequacy of oxygen delivery is assessed by sampling blood from the venous drainage line because this represents mixed venous oxygenation with the aim of maintaining venous saturations in excess of 75 per cent. In both types of support, it is important not to look at any of these parameters in isolation but instead to look at all markers of the adequacy of perfusion such as lactate, acid-base balance, urine output and tissue perfusion.

The size of the oxygenator is matched to the patient and flow rate such that it is capable of achieving 95 per cent oxygen saturation of the blood leaving the oxygenator. To increase oxygen delivery further, the haemoglobin can be raised and should be maintained in excess of 13 g/dL. In VAECMO, increasing blood flow rates also increases the rate of delivery of oxyhaemoglobin to the tissues. In VVECMO, higher pump flow rates may also deliver more oxyhaemoglobin to the patient, but they also may result in more re-circulation with a net reduction in true delivery to the patient. Carbon dioxide removal occurs in the membrane oxygenator via diffusion from the higher blood concentration across the membrane to the very low CO_2 concentration in the gases used to 'ventilate' the oxygenator. To improve efficiency, the blood and air phases pass in opposing directions to reduce the effect of a potential equilibrium. To increase CO_2 removal, the rate or 'sweep' of glass flow through the oxygenator should be increased.

In VAECMO

To *increase* O_2 delivery,
- Increase haemoglobin.
- Increase pump blood flow.

To *decrease* CO_2,
- Increase flow of gases through oxygenator ('sweep')

There is a wide range in the average length of circulatory support, but there is agreement that the longer the period of support, the worse is the outcome. In VAECMO for cardiac recovery after surgery, the absence of any ventricular function by 72 hours is a poor prognostic sign. Most survivors will have recovered after eight to ten days of support. Several groups have reported an association between the need for renal supportive therapy during ECMO and early death, but with a trend towards more aggressive early haemofiltration to correct blood chemistry, this is no longer an accurate predictor. Once stable, any patient who is placed on support after cardiac surgery should have a cardiac catheter within the first 48 to 72 hours to ensure that there aren't any correctable cardiac lesions that may be precluding recovery. VVECMO for respiratory failure is usually associated with longer periods of support, but this depends upon the presenting pathology.

ECMO for Cardiopulmonary Resuscitation (ECPR)

There are increasing reports and experiences using emergency ECMO during refractory cardiopulmonary arrest, especially following cardiac surgery. The ELSO Registry in 2012 identified 2,346 reported paediatric cases of ECPR with a survival to discharge of 39 per cent in neonates and 40 per cent in children. It is likely that all these children would have died without support. With rapid deployment of ECPR following a witnessed cardiac arrest in association with effective interim cardiac massage and systemic cooling, there is a relatively low associated morbidity. In an attempt to reduce the time to initiation of ECMO, units are maintaining wet primed circuits with designated teams and emergency activation protocols. The fastest situation is to have a resident ECMO team permanently within the hospital, but for the majority of units, this is not currently feasible.

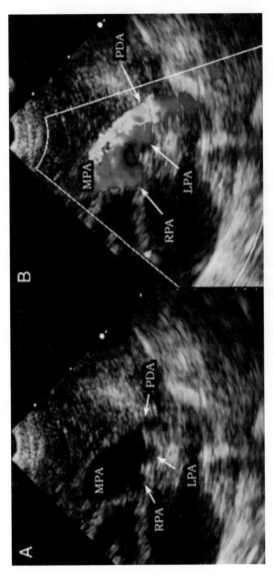

Figure 5.1 Echo images of a moderate-sized PDA and the trifurcating vies of the main and branch pulmonary arteries.

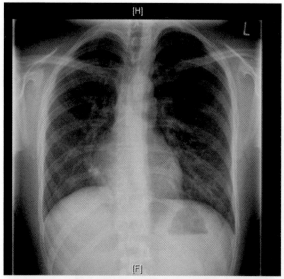

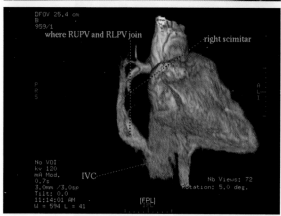

Figure 8.3 CXR and MRI reconstruction in scimitar syndrome showing the right pulmonary veins draining thought the 'scimitar' channel to the IVC.

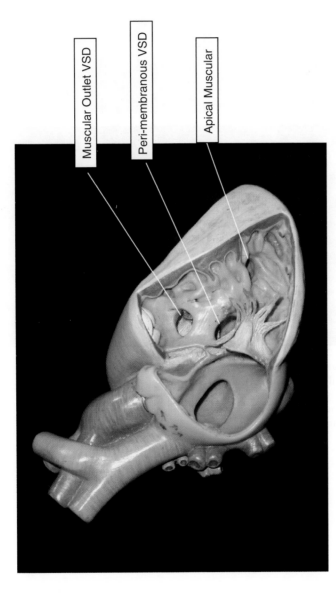

Muscular Outlet VSD

Peri-membranous VSD

Apical Muscular

Figure 9.1 3D model of the heart with the free wall of the right atrium and ventricle removed. Arrows show the positions of commonly occurring VSDs.

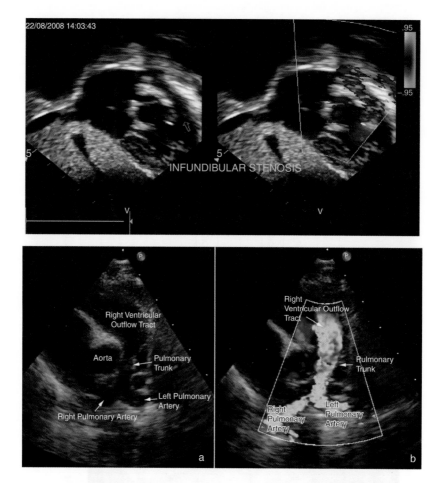

Figure 11.3 Echocardiographic still images of tetralogy of Fallot showing turbulent flow in the long, narrowed right ventricular infundibulum. The lower two images (A and B) show the composite hypoplasia of small infundibulum, valve annulus, and main and branch pulmonary arteries.

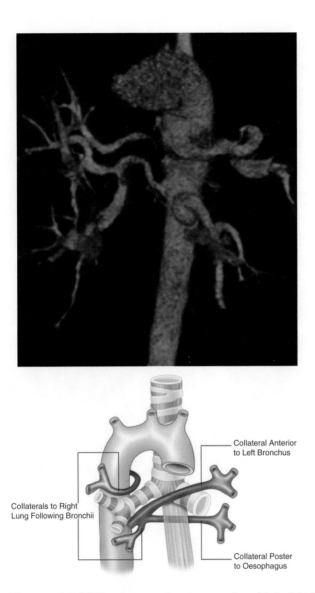

Figure 12.2 MRI reconstructive image of multiple MAPCAs and diagram demonstrating the relationship of MPACAs to the major airways and the oesophagus.

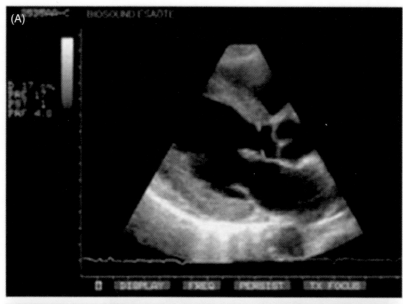

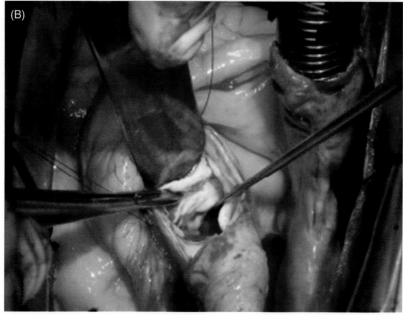

Figure 14.1 Echo image of (A) discrete sub-aortic membrane and (B) operative view through the aortic valve.
Source: From Kratiochvil F et al. Cor et Vasa Volume 59, Issue 5, October 2017, Pages e436–e440.

Pre- Banding: severe TR   Post- Banding: septum splinted
                                            reduction in TR

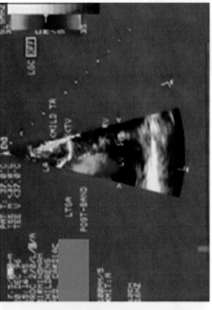

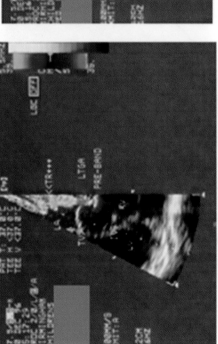

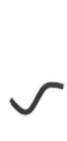

Figure 15.2 Echo images focusing on the position of the interventricular septum of a patient with ccTGA before and after PA banding. The shape of the septum changes from S-shaped to a straighter configuration, as emphasized by the solid lines below the images.

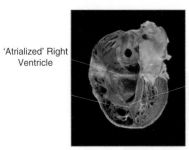

'Atrialized' Right
Ventricle

Apical Displacement of
the Tricuspid Valve

Figure 15.3 Ebstein's anomaly. The apical displacement of the tricuspid valve is clearly shown, creating a large 'atrialized' portion of the RV. The inferior leaflet of the TV is plastered along the free wall of the heart with multiple fibro-muscular connections, described as failed delamination of the valve.
Source: From Warnes CA et al. Journal of the American College of Cardiology : Volume 54, Issue 21, 17 November 2009, Pages 1903–1910.

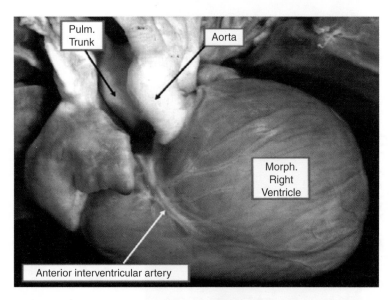

Figure 18.1 Heart with congenitally corrected transposition.
Source: Courtesy of Anderson R, *Cardiac Morphology*.

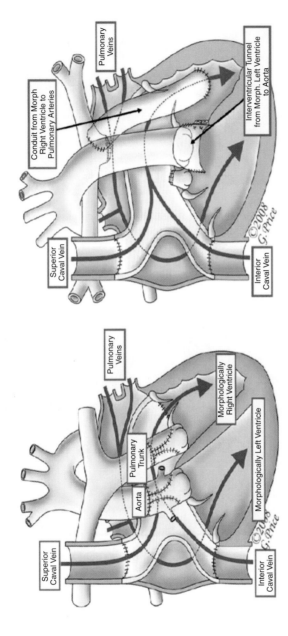

Figure 18.2 (A) Double-switch procedure in ccTGA. (B) Rastelli-Senning procedure in ccTGA.
Source: Courtesy of Anderson R, *Cardiac Morphology*.

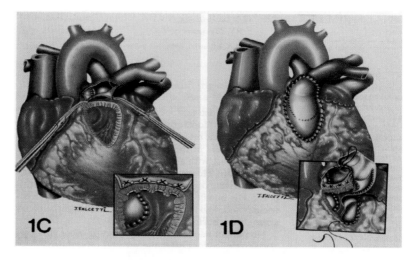

Figure 19.3 Direct anastomosis of the pulmonary arteries to the ventriculotomy. The defect is then roofed over with a patch, avoiding the need for a valved conduit.
Source: From Barbero-Marcial et al. A technique for correction of truncus arteriosus types I and II without extracardiac conduits. *Journal Thoracic Cardiovascular Surgery* 1990; 99: 364–69.

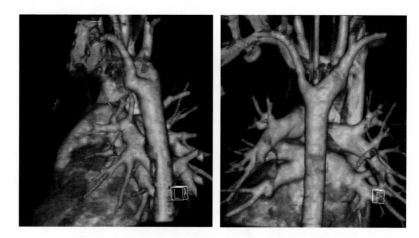

Figure 22.4 MRI reconstruction showing a right-sided arch with anomalous left subclavian artery arising from a diverticulum of Kommerell. The ductal ligament will insert into the base of the diverticulum but does not show on the MRI.

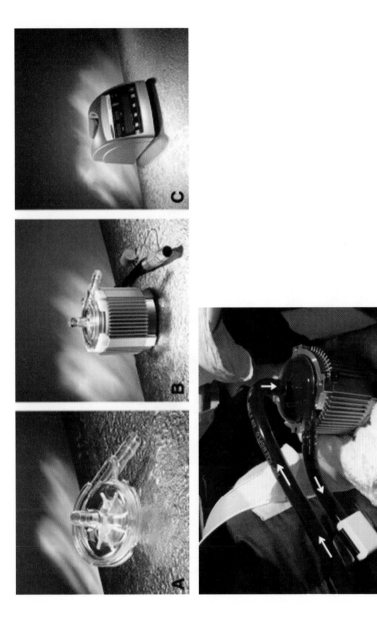

Figure 26.1 Levotronix rotating magnet system, which can be used for ECMO or for ventricular assist. (A) shows the pump head, (B) the pump head fitted into the magnetic housing and (C) the drive unit that controls rotation speed. The last image shows the system in use with the inlet an outlet pipes identified with arrows.
Source: Stainback RF et al. Journal of Thoracic and Cardiovascular Surgery Volume 141, Issue 4, April 2011, Pages 932–939, Ranjit J et al and Journal of the American Society of Echocardiography Volume 28, Issue 8, August 2015, Pages 853–909.

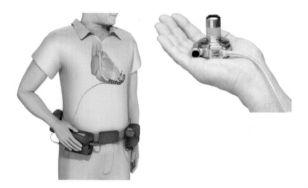

Figure 26.2 Heartware implantable assist device.
Source: From Horvath V et al. *Cor et Vasa* Volume 57, Issue 2, April 2015, Pages e70–e74.

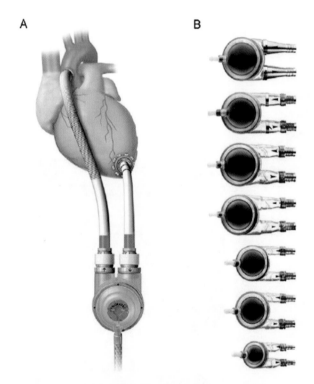

Figure 26.3 External VAD systems for circulatory support: (A) The Thoratec System and (B) The Berlin Heart in its various sizes.
Source: From Hehir DA et al. *World J Pediatr Congenit Heart Surg.* 2012 Jan 1;3(1):58–66.

Chapter 25

Surgery for Adult Congenital Heart Disease

David J. Barron

Introduction

An increasingly quoted statistic in recent times is the statement that there are now more adults alive with congenital heart disease than there are children. This reflects the fact that paediatric and neonatal cardiac surgery outcomes have transformed the natural history of these conditions. Fifty years ago, 85 per cent of all complex congenital heart conditions were lethal in childhood, whereas now over 85 per cent would be expected to survive into adulthood.

However, this survival does not come without cost, and many patients will have residual lesions or develop new problems related to their underlying condition and previous surgery. Consequently, the area of adult congenital heart disease (sometimes also known as 'grown-up congenital heart disease' (GUCH)) has become a rapidly expanding field with the need for surgical as well as expert cardiology care. The indications for surgery in these patients can be broadly divided into three categories:

1. *Newly diagnosed congenital heart disease in adulthood.* These are most commonly atrial septal defects (ASDs), partial atrio-ventricular septal defects (AVSDs) or lesser degrees of coarctation that have never presented during childhood and are picked up due to the development of symptoms or a chance finding on examination. Alternatively, progression of known lesions from childhood such as a dysplastic aortic valve may become clinically significant later in life and require a first intervention in adulthood.

2. *The residua and sequelae of procedures performed during childhood.* This is by far the largest group and includes replacing conduits and valves placed during childhood due to degeneration or outgrowth. It also includes the progression of pulmonary regurgitation following repair of Fallot's tetralogy leading to the need for pulmonary valve replacement (see below) or the progression of left ventricular outflow tract stenosis after the Rastelli procedure. Residual lesions include residual ASDs following childhood repair or valvar regurgitation after AVSD repair.

3. *Problems arising from the natural history of the underlying conditions or previous procedures.* This includes such conditions as ascending aortic dilatation in pulmonary atresia/tetralogy of Fallot and in the post-Ross procedure and right atrial dilatation following the Fontan procedure necessitating conversion to total cavo-pulmonary connection.

A summary of the frequency of ACHD procedures is shown in Table 25.1.

Special Considerations in ACHD Surgery

The median age for these procedures is still in the mid-twenties; thus, although there are increasing numbers of older patients, this is still mainly a population of young adults. Consequently, the choice of valve replacements and conduits has to reflect both the need for longevity

Table 25.1 Case Mix of Adult Congenital Surgical Procedures

Pulmonary valve replacement	25–38%
Secundum ASD	15–25%
Partial AVSD	5–7%
Aortic valve replacement/Ross	5–7%
Conduit replacement	4–6%
Sinus venosus ASD	6–8%
Ebstein's tricuspid repair/replacement	4–5%
Reoperation on Mustard/Senning	2–4%
Coarctation repair	2%
Fontan Revision	2%
VSD	3%
Palliative procedures – shunts and Glenn	3%

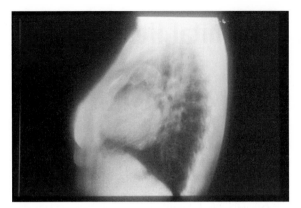

Figure 25.1 Lateral CXR of a patient who has previously undergone repair of pulmonary atresia using a homograft conduit. The conduit has become densely calcified and can be adherent to the back of the sternum at re-operation.

and the expectations of young adults, particularly women and the issues of pregnancy. In terms of the procedures themselves, over 70 per cent are re-operations with the attendant risks of redo – sternotomy and possible need for femoral bypass. Patients may also already have undergone multiple previous procedures, which can make surgery technically difficult with densely adherent structures and stiff and calcified old conduits and patchwork. Previous homografts can become densely calcified and adherent to the chest wall (Figure 25.1), making sternotomy hazardous. This highlights the importance of protective measures taken at the original procedure, such as the placement of membranes behind the sternum and partial closure of the pericardium.

Drug compliance and lifestyle are important considerations, as is the risk that bioprosthetic valves are likely to last for shorter periods due to active use. Thus, there is a strong focus on valve repair and reconstruction where possible.

Pulmonary Valve Replacement

The commonest procedure in ACHD surgery is pulmonary valve replacement in adults who underwent repair of tetralogy of Fallot in childhood. Most patients would have received a trans-annular patch, laying open the pulmonary valve at the time of initial repair. The pulmonary regurgitation is well tolerated throughout childhood, but the chronic volume load leads to progressive right ventricular dilatation, which, in turn, leads to exercise intolerance as the ventricle becomes less compliant with age and distension (Figure 25.2). There has been increasing concern

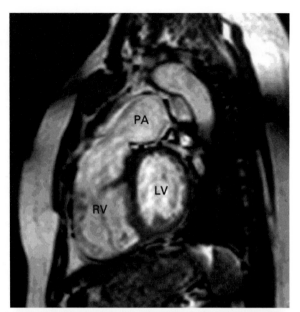

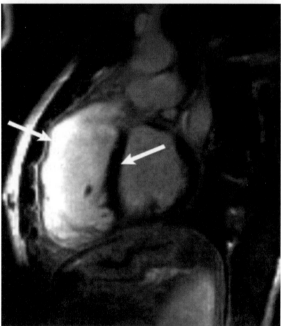

Figure 25.2 MRI showing dilated right ventricle and large right outflow tract in an adult patient who had previously undergone Fallot repair with a trans-annular patch (PA = pulmonary artery; RV = right ventricle; LV = left ventricle). The arrows show the degree of dilation of the right outflow tract.

that pulmonary valve replacement is being performed too late and that irreversible right ventricular injury can occur from allowing dilatation to go unchecked. A similar lesson has been learnt to that of aortic valve replacement in regurgitant disease, in that valve replacement is recommended based on ventricular dimensions rather than necessarily awaiting for symptoms. Measuring the absolute volume of the RV can be difficult due to its asymmetrical shape, but MRI has now provided accurate volume measurement. Valve replacement can now be recommended based on volumes reaching 140 to 150 mL/m^2 and/or evidence of reduced VO$_{2,max}$ on exercise testing. As further studies come to light, even these figures are being questioned, and replacement at a volume of 120 mL/m^2 has been suggested, with all RVs in this group returning to normal dimension during follow-up. Similar studies have also focused on right ventricular end-systolic volume, suggesting 85 mL/m^2 as a discriminant value. Tricuspid regurgitation is less common and usually is secondary to right ventricular dilatation. It usually can be successfully treated with annuloplasty with or without a valve ring at time of pulmonary valve replacement.

Surgery is safe, with peri-operative mortality of 1 to 2 per cent, and the valves most commonly used are bioprostheses. This avoids the need for anti-coagulation, and the expectation is that the bioprostheses will last longer than in the systemic circulation because the opening and closing forces on the valve are less. Current outcomes support this theory, with freedom from valve degeneration of 95 per cent at 10 years. Percutaneous pulmonary valve replacement is an attractive option for this group of patients – however, the technology is limited by the maximum size of the available valves (currently 22 mm) and the requirement for a solid 'landing zone' for the prosthesis. The majority of repaired Fallots have a giant outflow tract that is too large for one of these valves; however, once a stented bioprosthesis (or homograft) is in place, it is hoped that these will offer a secure site for placement of a percutaneous valve in the future. Devices are being developed with a 'cage' design that may enable valve placement in larger outflow tracts.

Other Important Areas

The Dilated Aorta. This is a common feature of many congenital conditions, particularly pulmonary atresia/tetralogy of Fallot and in the (neo-) aorta following arterial switch procedure. Dilatation is commoner in patients who had definitive repair at a later age and those who were initially palliated with arterial shunts. It is also commoner in males than in females. Although dilatation is common, the majority is not

of clinical significance, and progression is usually slow with minimal risk of rupture or dissection. Thus, management tends to be conservative, and most evidence favours medical treatment and regular surveillance for aortas of 45 to 55 mm. Surgery is also relatively conservative, with a role for ascending aortoplasty in moderate dilatation, and most interventions are usually performed 'incidentally' in that the primary indication for surgery has been pulmonary valve replacement or conduit replacement. Nevertheless, a root size of greater than 60 mm remains an absolute indication for root replacement (valve sparing, if possible).

Ebstein Surgery. This tricuspid valve anomaly with 'atrialization' of the RV due to apical displacement of the dysplastic tricuspid valve may not present (or be referred) until adulthood. Patients have severe tricuspid regurgitation but may tolerate this for many years without intervention; surgery has often been delayed until patients become symptomatic – by which time many have significant right ventricular dysfunction. There has been increasing interest in reconstructive techniques to repair these valves, particularly the 'cone' procedure, which has encouraging results. Most cases in adulthood also require placement of an annuloplasty ring as part of the repair. Atrial flutter is common, and concomitant right atrial maze is usually performed. These patients can be very challenging to manage postoperatively with resistant low cardiac output, and there may occasionally be a role for a bidirectional Glenn procedure together with valve repair to offload the failing right ventricle. Referral before right ventricular function deteriorates significantly (ejection fraction <45 per cent) and before left ventricular dysfunction develops may improve outcomes. Tricuspid valve replacement may be necessary in severe cases, and bioprosthetic valves are most commonly used with an 80 per cent freedom from re-operation at 10 to 15 years. Long-term outcome depends more on underlying right ventricular function than on whether the valve is repaired or replaced.

Fontan Conversion. The original Fontan procedures ('atrio-pulmonary connection') left the right atrium exposed to high venous pressures. Chronic exposure to these high pressures leads to distension of the atrium with stasis of blood within it and the risk of clot formation. Furthermore, the distension can lead to atrial arrhythmias, particularly flutter, which is often poorly tolerated. Thirdly, the distended atrium can also compress the left pulmonary veins, obstructing the Fontan circuit. Development of these complications can necessitate conversion to the 'modern' Fontan circulation, i.e. total cavopulmonary connection, which excludes the atrium from the high-pressure circulation and combines a right-sided maze procedure to control the atrial flutter. This is a major surgical undertaking, and it is important that the underlying ventricular function is well preserved and that pulmonary vascular resistance is still low to minimize surgical risk. Resternotomy in these patients with high venous pressures and a hugely dilated right atrium can be hazardous, and femoral bypass is usually necessary.

Transplantation. As the population of ACHD patients increases, there are greater numbers of cases being referred for transplantation with end-stage heart failure. The most difficult group of patients comprises those with Fontan circulations with a failing ventricle, and this group is only likely to increase as the cohorts of successfully treated children now grow into adulthood. Adult congenital patients can offer many challenges for the transplant surgeon; conditions with unusual venous connections or abnormal position of the heart can require detailed technical planning and modifications. Mobilization of the recipient's heart and creative options to make the necessary venous connections may require a joint approach with the 'congenital' surgeon and the transplant surgeon. Outcomes for heart transplantation for congenital heart disease are generally worse than those for cardiomyopathy or ischaemic heart disease. Early mortality is 10 to 15 per cent, which is partly due to the complexity of the surgery, but there is also a higher incidence of pulmonary vascular disease (particularly in the functionally univentricular circulations) in these patients, and the previous procedures and use of homografts can lead to raised panel-reactive antibodies (PRAs) that limit the donor pool and increase the risk of rejection. However, patients safely through the early stages have slightly better long-term survival than other groups. Combined with the problems of donor availability and the fact that more 'straightforward' cases with lower PRA may take priority, the total number of heart transplants performed for congenital heart disease is only 2 to 4 per cent of all transplants worldwide.

Acquired Disease

As the ACHD population continues to age, there is an increased likelihood of acquired heart disease (particularly coronary artery disease) occurring together with their congenital indications. Each component has to be treated on its own merits, but, as surgeons become increasingly specialized, there is a role for joint teams operating on these patients with surgeons expert in CABG working with the ACHD surgeons.

Controversies. The timing for surgical intervention remains an area for debate over a wide range of conditions: particularly in pulmonary valve replacement, where the thresholds for surgery are generally coming down, and surgery is being recommended earlier in the natural history. The same applies in Ebstein's anomaly, where there are the benefits of operating before right ventricular function deteriorates. There is an increasing use of tissue valves, recognizing the benefits of avoiding anti-coagulation in the young but accepting the need for further re-operations. Coarctation surgery has rapidly reduced with the advent of aortic stenting and is now rarely ever performed in adults. The future role for percutaneous pulmonary valves was discussed earlier. Atrial tachyarrhythmias are common in many of these patients, and there is a clear role for arrhythmia surgery – although the extent of the lesion set required and the role of a prophylactic maze is unknown. Despite the rapid progress in interventional stenting and percutaneous valves, it must be remembered that this is a young group of patients, and the long-term performance of these devices is unknown and provides further challenges for surgeons in the future. The adult population with a Fontan circulation will pose particular challenges, and long-term mechanical support devices may be a future option where transplantation is likely to be limited.

Further Reading

British Cardiac Society Working Party. Grown-up congenital heart (GUCH) disease: current needs and provision of service for adolescents and adults with congenital heart disease in the UK. *Heart* 2002; **88**(Suppl 1): i1–i14.

Khambadkone S, Coats L, Taylor A et al. Percutaneous pulmonary valve implantation in humans: results in 59 consecutive patients. *Circulation* 2005; **112**: 1189–97.

Mongeon FP, Gurvitz MZ, Broberg CS et al. Aortic root dilatation in adults with surgically repaired tetralogy of

Fallot: a multicenter cross-sectional study. Alliance for Adult Research in Congenital Cardiology (AARCC). *Circulation* 2013; **127**(2): 172–79.

Oosterhof T, van Straten A, Vliegen HW et al. Preoperative thresholds for pulmonary valve replacement in patients with corrected tetralogy of Fallot using cardiovascular magnetic resonance. *Circulation* 2007; **116**(5): 545–51.

Perloff JK, Warnes CA. Challenges posed by adults with repaired congenital heart disease. *Circulation* 2001; **103**: 2637–43.

Silversides CK, Marelli A, Beauchesne L et al. Canadian Cardiovascular Society 2009 Consensus Conference on the management of adults with congenital heart disease: executive summary. *Can J Cardiol* 2010; **26**(3): 143–50.

Therrien J, Siu SC, McLaughlin PR et al. Pulmonary valve replacement in adults late after repair of tetralogy of Fallot: are we operating too late? *J Am Coll Cardiol* 2000; **36**: 1670–75.

Vida VL, Berggren H, Brawn WJ et al. Risk of surgery for congenital heart disease in the adult: a multicentered European Study Alliance for Adult Research in Congenital Cardiology (AARCC). *Circulation* 2013; **127** (2): 172–79.

Chapter 26

Transplantation for Congenital Heart Disease

Phil Botha

Introduction

Although nearly half of all of children undergoing heart transplantation at present have developed end-stage cardiac failure due to intrinsic disease of the myocardium, the proportion undergoing transplantation for congenital heart disease (CHD) has gradually declined as techniques of repair have improved. A slowly increasing percentage of young adults with corrected or palliated CHD will, however, ultimately develop end-stage cardiac failure for which the only long-term therapy at present remains heart transplantation. Limited donor availability limits the application of this therapy and requires increasingly complex strategies to bridge these young patients to transplantation and maximize the use of available organs. There is growing concern that the increasing number of young adults with palliated single-ventricle circulations will exacerbate the shortage of donor organs with few available alternatives to improve their quality of life. Transplantation in young patients with a failing Fontan circulation provides a formidable challenge to the transplant team, not least because of the deleterious effects of long-term raised venous pressure and cyanosis on hepatic, haematological and renal function but also the impact that cardiac debilitation can have on the course immediately after transplantation. Multiple previous surgeries often lead to severe mediastinal adhesions and immune sensitization, which increase both the operative and logistical complexities of the transplantation procedure.

Anatomy

Very few anatomical barriers remain to preclude transplantation in CHD. Perhaps the most challenging, situs inversus, can be overcome by careful preoperative planning and the harvest of as much additional donor tissue as possible to aid reconstruction. Limiting the graft warm ischaemic time similarly requires careful planning,

completing in-situ reconstruction of the great veins and arteries where required prior to the onset of warm ischaemia. Perhaps the only anatomical features that render transplantation not feasible are extensive stenoses of the pulmonary arteries or veins beyond the area amenable to surgical repair. Heart-lung transplantation is often the only viable therapy under these circumstances. The small number of paediatric heart-lung transplants performed worldwide each year (only five to 10 paediatric heart-lung transplants are reported to the International Society for Heart and Lung Transplantation every year) reflects the extreme scarcity of suitable donor organ blocks and the relatively lower survival in this patient group (see 'Outcomes').

Immunology

As with all other cardiac transplants, blood type and weight are the major determinants of donor availability. In children younger than 2 years of age, however, the development of antibodies to the major ABO blood group antigens is incomplete, and during this period, ABO-incompatible cardiac transplantation has been undertaken with good results and the development of long-term immune tolerance to the non-self ABO antigens. Full blood-volume exchange transfusion is usually undertaken intra-operatively, and close postoperative monitoring for the development of increasing levels of anti-graft antibodies and antibody-mediated rejection is instituted. Previous blood transfusions and homograft material used in cardiac and vascular reconstructions frequently cause sensitization to HLA antigens in patients with CHD. The panel-reactive antibody (PRA) test is undertaken at transplant assessment to ascertain the levels of antibodies to common HLA antigens. Patients sensitized to more than 75 per cent of common major HLA antigens often face very protracted waiting periods on the transplant list and the possibility of not finding a suitable donor in time. The use of anti-CD20 antibody serum seems to reduce the development of

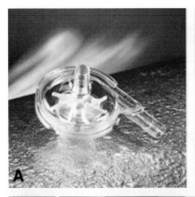
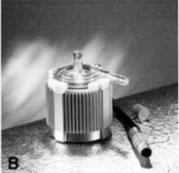
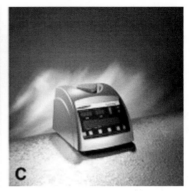
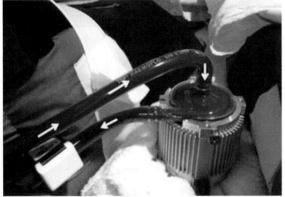

Figure 26.1 Levotronix rotating magnet system, which can be used for ECMO or for ventricular assist. (A) shows the pump head, (B) the pump head fitted into the magnetic housing and (C) the drive unit that controls rotation speed. The last image shows the system in use with the inlet an outlet pipes identified with arrows.
Source: Stainback RF et al. Journal of Thoracic and Cardiovascular Surgery Volume 141, Issue 4, April 2011, Pages 932–939, Ranjit J et al and Journal of the American Society of Echocardiography Volume 28, Issue 8, August 2015, Pages 853–909.
(A black-and-white version of this figure will appear in some formats. For the colour version, please refer to the plate section.)

activated plasma cells producing injurious antibodies. The logistics of donor preparation and organ procurement, along with the relatively short tolerated ischaemic time of the cardiac allograft, prevents prospective cross-matching to reduce the deleterious effects of a positive cross-match on rejection and graft longevity.

Mechanical Circulatory Support (MCS)

Internationally, around a third of paediatric heart transplant patients reported to the International Society for Heart and Lung Transplantation (ISHLT) are bridged to transplantation by MCS. The relatively small number of children requiring treatment for end-stage cardiac failure and the wide variation in required pump output for different-sized children have resulted in the development of paediatric MCS lagging behind that for adults by a considerable margin. Pulsatile extra-corporeal devices have been abandoned in adult practice in favour of continuous-flow pumps

with a resulting marked reduction in morbidity and the emergence of durable support options that enable destination therapy in those not suitable for transplantation. In children, however, the Berlin Heart extra-corporeal pump remains the only device presenting options for support of patients from neonatal to adult size for more than 30 days through a range of pumps from 10 to 50 mL (Figure 26.1). This has proven considerably more durable than ECMO, which until the 1980s was the only modality suitable to provide MCS to children. The modern ECMO devices such as the rotating levitated magnetic systems have proven to be well tolerated for prolonged periods of extra-corporeal support as a bridge to transplantation and are increasingly used as a short-term bridge in acute situations (Figure 26.2). In recent years, implantable continuous-flow pumps have increasingly been used in children with improving results. This has proven feasible in paediatric patients

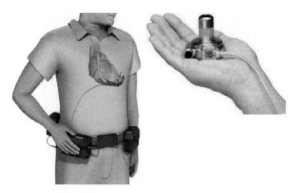

Figure 26.2 Heartware implantable assist device.
Source: From Horvath V et al. *Cor et Vasa* Volume 57, Issue 2, April 2015, Pages e70–e74.
(A black-and-white version of this figure will appear in some formats. For the colour version, please refer to the plate section.)

A   B

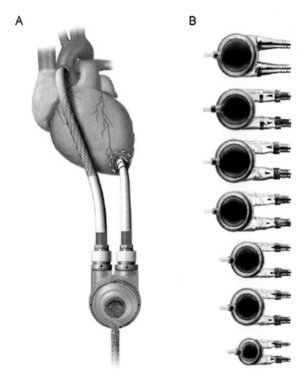

Figure 26.3 External VAD systems for circulatory support: (A) The Thoratec System and (B) The Berlin Heart in its various sizes.
Source: From Hehir DA et al. *World J Pediatr Congenit Heart Surg.* 2012 Jan 1;3(1):58–66.
(A black-and-white version of this figure will appear in some formats. For the colour version, please refer to the plate section.)

down to a weight of 13 kg and in many anatomical substrates, including the systemic right ventricle and failing single-ventricle circulation. Smaller, more durable pumps are eagerly awaited, with the Jarvik 2015 pump and Heartware devices

recently re-entering clinical trials (Figure 26.3). These systems still require an external drive line, but tunnelling these lines has reduced the risk of line infection, and rapid improvement in battery technology has provided increasingly portable battery packs.

Transplantation Surgery

Donor Selection

The scarcity of donor organs has led to a relaxation of once-strict donor selection criteria and the increasing use of 'marginal donors' not deemed suitable in earlier time periods. Typically, paediatric donors do not, however, have co-morbidities that can have a detrimental effect on post-transplantation function, such as systemic hypertension, atherosclerosis and smoking history. It has been repeatedly shown that selection criteria have been unnecessarily strict in the past and that many organs have gone to waste that could potentially have been used for successful heart transplantation. The donor echocardiogram can demonstrate signs of myocardial dysfunction secondary to the injurious effects of brain stem death, which will often reverse after transplantation. The presence of varying degrees of pulmonary hypertension in the CHD population requires the use of only good-quality donor organs, and the small size of the recipients excludes many adult donors. It is best to avoid the use of an under-sized donor in the setting of pulmonary hypertension, as it is thought that a slightly over-sized donor is protective against right ventricular dysfunction in the early post-transplant phase. The lower availability of very small donors also necessitates the use of size-mismatched donors, and over-sizing to 200 per cent of body weight in smaller children is generally considered to be safe.

Coordination

Good communication is paramount in achieving successful transplantation in CHD. The multi-organ retrieval team needs to work in concert to complete their respective organ assessments, dissection and finally organ explant after application of the aortic cross-clamp and administration of organ preservation solutions. Often the congenital cardiac recipient is the rate-limiting step to proceed with organ procurement for all teams involved because of the long time required for re-operative sternotomy after multiple previous surgeries and possibly mechanical circulatory support and the limitation of graft ischaemia preferably to below 4 hours. Early assessment of cardiac function and donor suitability by the cardiac team is critical, as this allows the implanting team to initiate recipient transfer to the operating room, anaesthesia, (often challenging) line placement and re-sternotomy. The retrieving surgeon, in the interim, needs to apply vigilance to prevent deterioration in the donor condition during prolonged dissection by the abdominal team and possibly delayed cross-clamping to allow recipient dissection to proceed to a safe point where implantation will not be delayed.

Careful planning for re-sternotomy should include cross-sectional thoracic imaging and Doppler assessment of peripheral arterio-venous patency. Many surgeons would prefer to complete re-sternotomy and dissection without instituting peripheral bypass, if possible, to limit the duration of cardiopulmonary bypass during prolonged dissection of adhesions and improve postoperative haemostasis. Additionally, the cardiopulmonary bypass setup can be prepared for full blood volume exchange on initiation of bypass in the setting of ABO-incompatible transplantation.

Reconstruction/Implantation

If extensive reconstruction of the central pulmonary arteries is required, this can be undertaken using Gore-Tex or homograft patch before the onset of warm ischaemia. Donor pulmonary artery can also be removed whilst maintaining cold preservation or directly implanted if less extensive reconstruction is required. In situs inversus, the atrial implantation can be achieved using a modification of the standard Lower-Shumway technique with the addition of an atrial baffle if required. A left superior vena cava (SVC) is preferably implanted to the donor brachiocephalic vein to avoid the need for a prosthetic conduit. If the inferior vena cava (IVC) is interrupted with hemi-azygous continuation to the left atrial roof, a tunnel to the right atrium is created using recipient atrium or donor pericardium. If the left

SVC drains via the coronary sinus, this can be preserved and incorporated into the right atrial anastomosis, with over-sewing of tributaries to the recipient heart. A baffle of recipient atrium can be sewn to the inferior recipient pericardium to allow re-implantation of a malpositioned left IVC to a normally positioned donor IVC.

Outcomes

Although early survival has improved significantly over the past three decades, long-term survival in children after heart transplantation remains limited by graft vasculopathy, malignancy and infection. Long-term survival in paediatric heart transplant recipients exceeds that of adults, with a median survival of 16 years. Children undergoing transplantation for CHD continue to be at higher risk of early mortality, although in the longer term outcomes match those of dilated cardiomyopathy. Single centres have demonstrated good outcomes in children transplanted for failing single-ventricle CHD, with higher early mortality in the adult group. Median survival after paediatric heart-lung transplantation in cases reported to the ISHLT remains disappointing at 2.4 years for CHD and 4.8 years for pulmonary hypertension.

Further Reading

De Rita F, Hasan A, Haynes S et al. Mechanical cardiac support in children with congenital heart disease with intention to bridge to heart transplantation. *Eur J Cardiothorac Surg* 2014; **46**(4): 656–62.

Henderson HT, Canter CE, Mahle WT et al. ABO-incompatible heart transplantation: analysis of the Pediatric Heart Transplant Study (PHTS) database. *J Heart Lung Transplant* 2012;**31**(2): 173–79.

Hosseinpour A-R, González-Calle A, Adsuar-Gómez A et al. Surgical technique for heart transplantation: a strategy for congenital heart disease. *Eur J Cardiothorac Surg* 2013; **44**(4): 598–604.

ISHLT.org: www.ishlt.org/registries/slides.asp? slides=heartLungRegistry.

Index